New Trends in Allergy and Atopic Eczema

Chemical Immunology and Allergy

Vol. 96

Series Editors

Johannes Ring Munich

Kurt Blaser Davos

Monique Capron Lille

Judah A. Denburg Hamilton

Stephen T. Holgate Southampton

Gianni Marone Naples

Hirohisa Saito Tokyo

New Trends in Allergy and Atopic Eczema

Volume Editors

Johannes Ring Munich
Ulf Darsow Munich
Heidrun Behrendt Munich

24 figures, 8 in color, and 6 tables, 2012

KARGER

Basel · Freiburg · Paris · London · New York · New Delhi · Bangkok · Beijing · Tokyo · Kuala Lumpur · Singapore · Sydney

Chemical Immunology and Allergy
Formerly published as 'Progress in Allergy' (Founded 1939),
continued 1990–2002 as 'Chemical Immunology'
Edited by Paul Kallós 1939–1988, Byron H. Waksman 1962–2002

Prof. Dr. med. Dr. phil. Johannes Ring
Prof. Dr. med. Ulf Darsow
Prof. Dr. med. Heidrun Behrendt
Klinik und Poliklinik für Dermatologie und
Allergologie am Biederstein
ZAUM - Zentrum Allergie und Umwelt
Technische Universität München
Christine Kühne Center of Allergy Research and
Education (CK-CARE)
Biedersteiner Strasse 29
DE–80802 Munich (Germany)
E-Mail johannes.ring@lrz.tum.de

Bibliographic Indices. This publication is listed in bibliographic services, including Current Contents® and PubMed/MEDLINE.

www.karger.com
Printed in Germany on acid-free and non-aging paper (ISO 9706) by Kraft Druck GmbH, Ettlingen
ISSN 1660–2242
e-ISSN 1662–2898
ISBN 978–3–8055–9894–1
e-ISBN 978–3–8055–9895–8

Contents

Preface

Allergy and allergic diseases have increased in prevalence dramatically over the last decades. Relevant determinants influencing the development of allergic inflammation come from the environment and are either enhancing – promoting allergy – or protective in nature. The lack of protective factors such as early stimulation of the immune system through infection or parasite infestation by improved hygiene seems to go along with allergy promoting effects of environmental pollutants such as traffic exhaust – fine or ultrafine particles – or tobacco smoke in the indoor air. Climate change with higher CO_2 concentrations in the atmosphere and increases in the Earth's surface temperature may contribute to an increase in allergic diseases by prolonging the flowering period of pollinating plants and immigration of allergenic neophytes.

Great progress has been made in elucidating the pathomechanisms of allergic reactions both at the level of molecular genetics and in the understanding of the complex orchestra of cells and mediators in the allergic inflammation.

It has become clear that not only the deviated immune response is a prerequisite for allergy with dominant Th2 reactions and consequent IgE production, but also the epithelial barrier is of crucial importance both in the mucosal surface of the airway and in the skin.

In spite of the great progress in the experimental allergology and immunology, there is still a tremendous gap between the theoretical knowledge and the practical performance in daily life treating allergic patients in the office or in the hospital. This becomes especially obvious when we think of subjective symptoms such as itch, which is the major symptom of allergic skin disease.

Only on the basis of a better understanding of the pathomechanisms and the molecular pathways involved can new therapeutic and preventive strategies for future management of allergic patients seem possible.

This volume brings together a carefully selected list of articles based upon lectures given at the International Symposium 'New Trends in Allergy VII' together with the '6th Georg Rajka Symposium on Atopic Dermatitis' organized in Munich in July 2010. At this symposium, two remarkable traditions were joined: the symposia 'New Trends in Allergy', which began in 1980 in Munich and have since been held in 5-year intervals in Munich, Hamburg and Davos. The International Symposium on

Atopic Dermatitis was started by Professor Georg Rajka in Oslo and held five times in Norway. Since 1996, taking the name of the founder, they have been continued all over the world, taking place in Aarhus, Davos, Portland, Rome, Arcachon, Kyoto and Munich, and have brought together all the experts both from clinics and research interested in the field of atopic eczema. The next Georg Rajka Symposium will be held in 2012 in Moshi, Tanzania, in order to stress the fact that allergy and eczema is not a disease of the so-called Western world, but can be found also in rural regions in central sub-Saharan Africa.

We would like to thank Alberto Giannetti (Modena), Alain Taïeb (Bordeaux), Kristian Thestrup-Petersen (Aarhus) and Hirohisa Takigawa (Matsumoto) for help in the development of the Rajka symposia. Mr. Preussler and Mrs. Burk deserve thanks for the excellent organization of the symposium in Munich. A final highlight was the performance of an 'allergy musical' by the coworkers of the Department of Dermatology and Allergy as well as the ZAUM [Zentrum Allergie und Umwelt (Center for Allergy and Environment)] at the Biederstein Campus of the Technische Universität München in the Löwenbräukeller: 'King Ludwig II – His Life, His Death, His Allergy!' In this play, undiscussed aspects of the mysterious end of Bavaria's dream king were put to stage in a humorous fashion, at the same time giving a new example of very well accepted allergy education.

Thanks also go to Mr. Nold and Mr. Brian from Karger Publishers for the excellent help in the production of this book.

We would also like to thank the Christine Kühne Center of Allergy Research and Education (CK-CARE) as well as the Munich Allergy Research Society (Verein zur Förderung der Forschung und Fortbildung auf dem Gebiet dermatologischer und allergologischer Erkrankungen e.V.) for their generous support.

Johannes Ring, Munich
Ulf Darsow, Munich
Heidrun Behrendt, Munich

Ring J, Darsow U, Behrendt H (eds): New Trends in Allergy and Atopic Eczema.
Chem Immunol Allergy. Basel, Karger, 2012, vol 96, pp 1–6

Allergy in Evolution

Thomas A.E. Platts-Mills

Asthma and Allergy Disease Center, University of Virginia, Charlottesville, Va., USA

Abstract

The 'foreignness' of proteins that we encounter in our homes and outdoors is in large part dependent on their evolutionary distance from man. This is relevant to understanding the differences between mammalian allergens, e.g. cats, and arthropod allergens, e.g. mites and cockroaches, as well as to understanding responses to a wide range of food allergens. On the other hand, allergic disease has gone through a major evolution of its own from a prehygiene state where there is minimal production of allergen-specific IgE, to the production of high-titer IgE, and then to the dramatic increase in asthma. The challenge is to understand how changes in both hygiene and lifestyle have contributed to the changes in allergic disease.

The title carries the inevitable ambiguity about whether we are concerned with the ways in which allergy has evolved or the relevance of evolution to allergic disease. We will assume that allergic disease has not had a significant effect on evolution and that the speed with which allergic disease has developed excludes significant changes in human genetic material as a cause of the increase. On the other hand, it is possible, and indeed likely, that the form of immunity that today improves the ability to recognize and respond to a small number of inhaled particles (i.e. atopy) has been a benefit in survival against the major epidemic diseases of the past, e.g. the plague, smallpox, influenza, malaria and tuberculosis. This chapter will focus on (1) the evolution of molecules that are relevant to allergic disease today and (2) the ways in which allergic disease has evolved in the last 100 years.

Evolution of Protein Structures

Many of the proteins that are recognized as allergens today come from protein families that can easily be traced back to the archaebacteria. Thus the overall structure of Der p 1 is similar to a human cathepsin and also to a thiol protease from *Staphylococcus aureus* [1]. Equally, the structure of the birch pollen allergen Bet v 1 can be traced back to bacterial proteins [2]. Breiteneder and his colleagues [3] have made an excellent case that the immunogenicity of the tropomyosins as food allergens can be directly related to their evolutionary distance from the great apes. The important concept is that over long periods of time, i.e. hundreds of millions of years, the same structure has been used for many different biological purposes. Although the structure retains a strong homology, the amino acids used to make up that structure change relatively rapidly, and it is the amino acids that define both the B and T cell epitopes. In general, proteins change progressively and after about 100 million years they will be immunologically 'foreign'. Thus, we have not been separate from other mammals, e.g. cats, dogs, cows and mice, long enough for all the proteins to be foreign [4]. Dr. Spitzauer [5] describes this elegantly with, 'IgE antibody responses to mammalian proteins, at the borderline between foreign and self'. There are some human proteins, e.g. Toll-like receptors (TLR), that have such high homology with mammalian proteins that it is difficult to induce an antibody response to them in the mouse. For this reason, chickens are often used to make monoclonal antibodies to human TLR [6]. We assume that the issues which are relevant to a mouse in recognizing and responding to a human protein are similar to the issues that are relevant to a human recognizing proteins from mice or other mammals. On the other hand, there can be changes in the expression of a protein or in the form of a carbohydrate glycosylation which mean that the relevant molecule is effectively foreign to man. This appears to be true for the cat protein Fel d 1, which does not have a human homologue and is an extremely important allergen. Similarly, the gene for the enzyme α_1, 3-galactosyl transferase became inactive in the old world monkeys and great apes, approximately 10 million years ago [7, 8]. This change allows humans and other great apes to make an IgG and IgE antibody response to this oligosaccharide [7, 9]. Interestingly, the IgG antibody response to α-gal is a natural antibody response present in almost all immunocompetent adults and is most likely induced by bacterial oligosaccharides. By contrast, the IgE response to α-gal develops most often in adults and is primarily induced by tick bites [10].

Many of the major sources of allergens have been separated from humans for hundreds of millions of years. Thus, mites and cockroaches separated from us approximately 600 million years ago. We have been separate from plants for at least 1,500 million years, and fungi for 1,200 million years. In some cases, different major groups within these kingdoms separated early, e.g. trees and grasses, while in other cases separation occurred more recently, e.g. species within the grasses or within the insects. These differences may be very important for cross-reactivity between different allergens. For example, dust mites show very little cross-reactivity with insects, but cross-react extensively with scabies mites. Equally, there is extensive cross-reactivity of allergens between different insects such as lady bugs and cockroaches [11]. With very long periods of separation, there are other major changes that have occurred. Most obviously, the full methylation of DNA occurred with the hagfish and lampreys [12]. Unmethylated DNA and in particular the CpG motif is a potent activator of TLR-9 which enhances immune responses to proteins delivered with it [13]. Going a little further back, many bacteria have complex lipopolysaccharides in their cell walls that can activate TLR-4 [14]. Mite fecal particles contain unmethylated DNA from both mites and bacteria, as well as lipopolysaccharide and the protein allergens [15, 16]. Thus, it is not surprising that mite fecal particles, cockroach debris or pollen grains are such potent causes of IgE antibody responses.

'Evolution' of Allergic Diseases: 1870–2000

Hay fever appeared as a disease of affluent people around 1870, shortly after the introduction of clean water, widespread wearing of shoes and control of helminth infections. By 1946 in New York and 1950 in London, hay fever was epidemic. By contrast, asthma, particularly among children, remained rare until 1960. The rise in asthma from 1960 to 2000 has been documented in many ways: repeated sampling of populations in the ISAAC studies, evidence for major increases in the numbers of patients receiving treatment and hospital admission data [17, 18]. Therefore, it is possible to ask two questions: (1) 'How did "cleanliness" lead to an increase in allergic disease, initially manifested as hay fever?' and (2) 'Why did the major increase in asthma in the USA and UK not start until 1960 if the relevant changes in hygiene were complete by 1920?'.

In Ghana and other developing countries, it is possible to observe changes that are relevant to 'hygiene' occurring within a country or even within a large town. In Kumasi, children in a school for relatively affluent children had increased asthma, a high prevalence of high-titer IgE antibodies to mite allergens and a highly significant correlation between IgE to mites and asthma [19]. By contrast, asthma was less common in a less affluent school within the same town; only low-titer IgE antibody to mite was found in the sera, and this showed no relationship to symptomatic wheezing or fall in peak flow after exercise [19, 20]. The real differences between the two areas in the town appear to be clean water, 'better' food supplies and 'better' homes because antihelminth treatment was common throughout the population of this town and not restricted to the affluent group [19]. Thus, it appears that changes in hygiene that can be achieved within a typical African city can result in a change to a Western model of allergy and asthma within a few years [19, 21].

If we ask what changes occurred in London and New York in 1960, they do not appear to be related to hygiene. There were changes in antibiotic use and in vaccination policy, but the changes in water and housing quality had occurred at least 40 years earlier [22]. On the other hand, major changes in lifestyle started in the 1950s with the introduction of addictive television for children. These changes have been followed by the rise in obesity and changes in diet, but most obviously by dramatic changes in the physical activity of children [23].

Conclusions

The development of allergic disease has roughly occurred over the last 100 years in Europe, Australasia, Japan and North America. However, in Africa and South America, it is possible to observe Western patterns of allergic disease developing in close physical and temporal proximity to what could be called prehygiene communities. This creates an opportunity to evaluate both the important features of the Western model of allergic disease and the environmental changes that are necessary to make the change. There is good evidence from many studies that close exposure to farm animals, helminth infection or recurrent gastrointestinal infection can 'prevent' the development of allergic disease. However, in reality most children living in rural communities in Ecuador, Northern Brazil or Kenya are exposed to all of these. Therefore, the change that leads to a truly Western model of disease may depend on what changes have already occurred and whether we are interested in allergic disease in general or asthma specifically [19, 21]. By using New Zealand, UK, Virginia, large cities in the USA or Sweden as examples of the Western model, it is clear that there is a high prevalence of high-titer IgE antibodies to the relevant allergens, i.e. dust mites, cockroaches or cats, and that these IgE antibodies are strongly associated with allergic disease, i.e. OR of 6 or higher.

The most common cause of IgE antibody responses is the inhalation of particles repeatedly over a long period of time. The relevant protein allergens are foreign and most of the common allergen sources have been evolutionarily separate from the primates for at least 600 million years. The only major exceptions among the inhalant allergens are mammalian danders, including cats, dogs and rodents. That there is a difference in the response to animal danders is undoubted. In many studies, it is clear that a large number of allergic individuals who live in a house with a cat do not become allergic to cat allergens. Many of these subjects make IgG and IgG_4 antibodies to Fel d 1 without IgE antibodies [24]. Overall, IgE responses to cats are less common and of lower titer; whether this is the reason why asthma is less common, i.e. ≤10%, in countries where cats or dogs are the major sources of allergen than in countries where mite allergens are dominant, i.e. 20–25%, is not clear [25]. However, it is clear that the increase in asthma throughout the Western world has been as small as 0.5–5% in some countries compared with 2–20% in others. With increasing evolutionary distance, proteins become more foreign and the particles include other substances that are potent TLR ligands. It is therefore no surprise that pollen grains, mold spores, cockroach debris and mite fecal particles can induce immune responses with very low overall exposure. For mammalian dander, the proteins are less foreign, but the quantitative exposure is higher, and the pattern of response to very high exposure is different. Despite these important differences in the nature of the allergens in our environment, it is important to remember that the evolution of allergic disease has occurred rapidly and has been dramatically influenced not only by changes in hygiene, but also by many other aspects of lifestyle.

Acknowledgement

This work was supported by NIH grant No. AI-20565.

References

1 Platts-Mills TAE, Woodfolk J: Allergens and their role in the allergic immune response. Immunol Rev 2011;242:51–68.

2 Radauer C, Lackner P, Breiteneder H: The Bet v 1 fold: an ancient, versatile scaffold for binding of large, hydrophobic ligands. BMC Evol Biol 2008;8: 286.

3 Jenkins JA, Breiteneder H, Mills EN: Evolutionary distance from human homologs reflects allergenicity of animal food proteins. J Allergy Clin Immunol 2007;120:1399–1405.

4 Platts-Mills TA: The role of indoor allergens in chronic allergic disease. J Allergy Clin Immunol 2007;119:297–302.

5 Spitzauer S: Allergy to mammalian proteins: at the borderline between foreign and self? Int Arch Allergy Immunol 1999;120:259–269.

6 Finlay WJ, Bloom L, Cunningham O: Optimized generation of high-affinity, high-specificity single-chain Fv antibodies from multiantigen immunized chickens. Methods Mol Biol 2011;681:383–401.

7 Macher BA, Galili U: The Galalpha1, 3Galbeta1, 4GlcNAc-R (alpha-Gal) epitope: a carbohydrate of unique evolutionary and clinical relevance. Biochim Biophys Acta 2008;1780: 75–88.

8 Koike C, Uddin M, Wildman DE, Gray EA, Trucco M, Starzl TE, Goodman M: Functionally important glycosyltransferase gain and loss during catarrhine primate emergence. Proc Natl Acad Sci USA 2007; 104:559–564.

9 Chung CH, Mirakhur B, Chan E, Le QT, Berlin J, Morse M, Murphy BA, Satinover SM, Hosen J, Mauro D, et al: Cetuximab-induced anaphylaxis and IgE specific for galactose-alpha-1,3-galactose. N Engl J Med 2008;358:1109–1117.

10 Commins S, James H, Kelly E, Pochan S, Workman L, Perzanowski M, Kocan K, Fahy J, Nganga L, Ronmark E, et al: The relevance of tick bites to the production of IgE antibodies to the mammalian oligosaccharide galactose-α-1,3-galactose. J Allergy Clin Immunol 2011;127:1286–1293.

11 Nakazawa T, Satinover SM, Naccara L, Goddard L, Dragulev BP, Peters E, Platts-Mills TA: Asian ladybugs (*Harmonia axyridis*): a new seasonal indoor allergen. J Allergy Clin Immunol 2007;119:421–427.

12 Tweedie S, Charlton J, Clark V, Bird A: Methylation of genomes and genes at the invertebrate-vertebrate boundary. Mol Cell Biol 1997;17:1469–1475.

13 Liu K, Anderson G, Bozinovski S: DNA vector augments inflammation in epithelial cells via EGFR-dependent regulation of TLR4 and TLR2. Am J Respir Cell Mol Biol 2008;39:305–311.

14 Eisenbarth SC, Piggott DA, Huleatt JW, Visintin I, Herrick CA, Bottomly K: Lipopolysaccharide-enhanced, Toll-like receptor 4-dependent T helper cell type 2 responses to inhaled antigen. J Exp Med 2002;196:1645–1651.

15 Tovey ER, Chapman MD, Platts-Mills TA: Mite faeces are a major source of house dust allergens. Nature 1981;289:592–593.

16 Satinover S, Hulse K, Carper H, Platts-Mills TAE, Woodfolk J: Are the pro-allergic properties of house dust mite allergen explained by the adjuvant effects of mite DNA? J All Clin Immunol 2007;119:S259.

17 Weinmayr G, Weiland SK, Bjorksten B, Brunekreef B, Buchele G, Cookson WO, Garcia-Marcos L, Gotua M, Gratziou C, van Hage M, et al: Atopic sensitization and the international variation of asthma symptom prevalence in children. Am J Respir Crit Care Med 2007;176:565–574.

18 Crater DD, Heise S, Perzanowski M, Herbert R, Morse CG, Hulsey TC, Platts-Mills TAE: Asthma hospitalization trends in Charleston, South Carolina, 1956 to 1997: twenty-fold increase among black children during a 30-year period. Pediatrics 2001; 108:E97.
19 Stevens W, Addo-Yobo E, Roper J, Woodcock A, James H, Platts-Mills TA, Custovic A: Differences in both prevalence and titre of specific immunoglobulin E among children with asthma in affluent and poor communities within a large town in Ghana. Clin Exp Allergy 2011, E-pub ahead of print.
20 Addo-Yobo EO, Woodcock A, Allotey A, Baffoe-Bonnie B, Strachan D, Custovic A: Exercise-induced bronchospasm and atopy in Ghana: two surveys ten years apart. PLoS Med 2007;4:e70.
21 Perzanowski MS, Ng'ang'a LW, Carter MC, Odhiambo J, Ngari P, Vaughan JW, Chapman MD, Kennedy MW, Platts-Mills TA: Atopy, asthma, and antibodies to Ascaris among rural and urban children in Kenya. J Pediatr 2002;140:582–588.
22 Armstrong GL, Conn LA, Pinner RW: Trends in infectious disease mortality in the United States during the 20th century. JAMA 1999;281:61–66.
23 Crater SE, Platts-Mills TA: Searching for the cause of the increase in asthma. Curr Opin Pediatr 1998; 10:594–599.
24 Platts-Mills TAE, Vaughan J, Squillace S, Woodfolk J, Sporik R: Sensitisation, asthma, and a modified Th2 response in children exposed to cat allergen: a population-based cross-sectional study. Lancet 2001;357:752–756.
25 Eder W, Ege MJ, von Mutius E: The asthma epidemic. N Engl J Med 2006;355:2226–2235.

Prof. Thomas A.E. Platts-Mills
Asthma and Allergy Disease Center, University of Virginia
PO Box 801355
Charlottesville, VA 22908 (USA)
Tel. +1 804 924 5917, E-Mail tap2z@virginia.edu

Ring J, Darsow U, Behrendt H (eds): New Trends in Allergy and Atopic Eczema.
Chem Immunol Allergy. Basel, Karger, 2012, vol 96, pp 7–14

Climate Change, Environment and Allergy

Heidrun Behrendt · Johannes Ring

ZAUM – Zentrum Allergie und Umwelt (Center for Allergy and Environment), Technische Universität München, and Department of Dermatology and Allergy Biederstein, Technische Universität München, Munich, Germany

Abstract

Climate change with global warming is a physicometeorological fact that, among other aspects, will also affect human health. Apart from cardiovascular and infectious diseases, allergies seem to be at the forefront of the sequelae of climate change. By increasing temperature and concomitant increased CO_2 concentration, plant growth is affected in various ways leading to prolonged pollination periods in the northern hemisphere, as well as to the appearance of neophytes with allergenic properties, e.g. *Ambrosia artemisiifolia* (ragweed), in Central Europe. Because of the effects of environmental pollutants, which do not only act as irritants to skin and mucous membranes, allergen carriers such as pollen can be altered in the atmosphere and release allergens leading to allergen-containing aerosols in the ambient air. Pollen has been shown not only to be an allergen carrier, but also to release highly active lipid mediators (pollen-associated lipid mediators), which have proinflammatory and immunomodulating effects enhancing the initiation of allergy. Through the effects of climate change in the future, plant growth may be influenced in a way that more, new and altered pollens are produced, which may affect humans.

Allergic diseases represent one of the major health problems in many countries of the world. They have increased dramatically in prevalence during the last 50 years [2, 3, 5, 30, 32, 34, 38, 40]. Today the estimate is that 10–20 % of adults suffer from at least one allergic disease, 15–40% are sensitized against aeroallergens and 5–20% of children suffer from atopic eczema [33]. The reasons for this increased prevalence of allergic diseases are only partly known. Apart from genetic predisposition, which can be clearly shown in family or twin studies, environmental influences also play a distinctive role.

Environment and Allergy

Allergic diseases are among the few diseases where the actual causal factors (i.e. the allergens) are to a great extent chemically characterized and available as recombinant

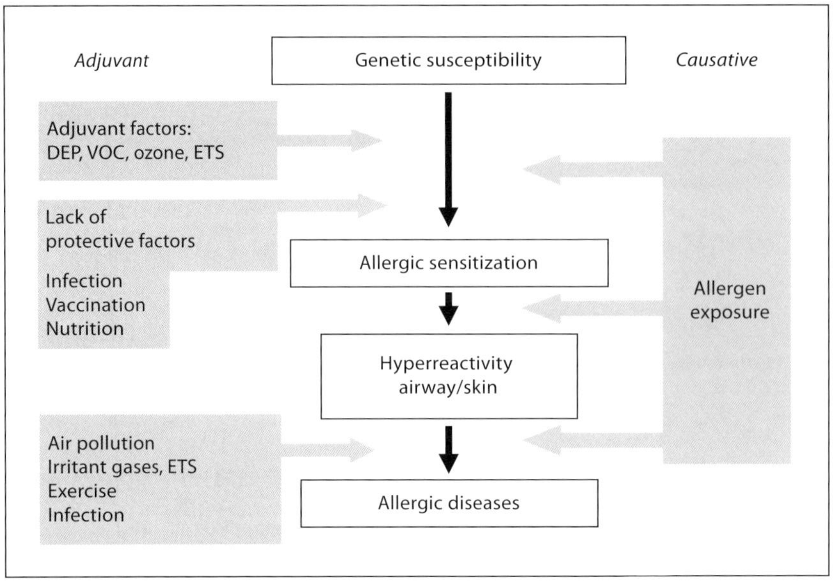

Fig. 1. Determinants of allergic inflammation (from [5, 6]).

proteins [32, 36]. The exposure to allergens is not only causal for the development of an allergic disease, but also for the elicitation of symptoms and the intensity of the actual clinical symptomatology. In the evaluation of environmental influences upon the development of allergies, the various levels of sensitization, skin or airway hyperreactivity, and manifest disease have to be differentiated [5, 6] (fig. 1).

There is no allergy without an allergen; this very simple fact is often forgotten when hypothetical concepts about the increase in allergen prevalence are discussed. It is without question that allergen exposure has changed over the last decades, both quantitatively and qualitatively. Regarding aeroallergens in indoor compartments, increased efforts to save energy have led to better insulated houses with increased growth of house dust mites in apartments. Furthermore, there is an increased tendency to having pets in rather small apartments in many countries of the world.

Environmental Pollution

Apart from causal-acting allergens, adjuvant factors from the environment play a role in the development of allergies. These factors may be either protective in nature, as infection stimuli of the immune system [9, 14, 15, 18, 28], or exert enhancing effects upon allergic sensitization and manifestation of allergic disease, such as environmental pollutants.

Environmental pollutants can be classified either according to the compartment (indoor vs. outdoor) [37], sources (fixed sources like industry emissions vs. mobile sources, e.g. traffic exhaust), or according to the production as primary pollutants which are directly released into the atmosphere (e.g. sulfur dioxide, nitrogen oxides, carbon monoxide, and particles) or secondary air pollutants which are only formed through chemical processes in the air (e.g. ozone).

There is evidence from epidemiological and experimental studies that several air pollutants are able to increase the risk of allergic diseases. Indoors, for example, substances from tobacco smoke exert allergy-enhancing effects both for allergic respiratory disease (rhinoconjunctivitis, asthma) and skin disease (atopic eczema) [19]. Outdoors, traffic exhaust seems to be the most important allergy-enhancing factor and is best characterized as fine or ultrafine particles [1, 13, 20, 23, 25, 26, 27, 29]. Experimental studies in animals have shown that exposure to fine and ultrafine particles – especially diesel exhaust particles – can increase susceptibility to IgE-mediated sensitization as well as intensity of clinical symptoms [1].

Western Lifestyle

From many epidemiological studies, it has become obvious that factors characterizing the 'Western' lifestyle are associated with increased allergy prevalence [31]. One socioeconomic factor is parental education, which is directly correlated to the prevalence of atopic diseases in the offspring. Another factor is family size: the number of siblings of an atopic child and, more generally, the number of people living in the same dwelling are all inversely correlated to the risk of developing an atopic disease. Furthermore, eating, living and entertaining habits may also need to be considered, e.g. children are spending more and more time in front of the TV and are thus spending less time with physical exercise outside (T. Platts-Mills, personal communication). Yet an additional factor is the increasing amount of calories in 'Western' food which can lead to obesity in children – there seems to be a positive correlation between BMI and the relative risk for developing asthma [11].

Climate Change

'Climate' represents the sum of atmospheric conditions and processes in spatial and temporal long-term distribution. In addition to the 'mean' of atmospheric conditions, the behavior over time and the variability of individual conditions and processes play a role. Every statement regarding climate is of a statistical nature and reflects longer periods of years, if not decades.

The surface of the Earth is heated by solar radiation, which leads to a natural greenhouse effect. Human activity can lead to an increase in the concentration of atmospheric greenhouse gases which adds to the natural effect in the sense of an additional anthropogenic greenhouse effect. Through the work of the Intergovernmental Panel Climate Change – which was awarded the Nobel Prize – it has become clear that in the last decades, the surface temperature of the Earth has increased to such a degree and so rapidly as never before seen in previously so-called cyclic changes of temperature [22]. The longest daily temperature measurements have been performed in Davos, Switzerland, where they have been recorded since the mid-19th century. Here the Physico-Meteorological Observatory Davos together with the World Radiation Center have been measuring the irradiation from the sun over the last 30 years and have found it to be decreasing. Therefore, the obvious increase in global temperature cannot be explained by altered solar irradiation, but has to be seen as being a result of anthropogenic activities.

Global warming is thus no myth or journalistic exaggeration, but a physicometeorological fact and represents an aspect of climate change which among others will also affect human health. One example of the effect of climate change on health was the extremely hot summer Europe experienced in 2003 and which went along with many fatalities due to heat, mostly in France. The seemingly increasing incidence of 'natural catastrophes' such as flooding, thunderstorms, etc., may also be a result of climate change.

Parameters of climate change seem to have both an enhancing as well as inhibitory effect upon UV irradiation on the Earth's surface. In a summarizing analysis, the Intergovernmental Panel Climate Change came to the conclusion that there is a slight increase in UV exposure through climate change, possibly leading to an increase in skin cancer and photodermatoses. With regard to human health, in addition to cardiovascular disease and infectious diseases, allergies seem to also be at the forefront of the adverse effects of climate change.

Climate Change Effects upon Pollen

Pollen not only can elicit allergic rhinoconjunctivitis and asthma in inducing symptoms in upper and lower airways, but can also exacerbate eczematous skin lesions in patients with atopic eczema. This has been shown by the 'atopy patch test' where the epicutaneous application of pollen grains upon normal untreated human skin was able to induce an eczematous inflammation [31]. Children with this type of pollen allergy also showed significantly associated increases in eczema symptomatology during high pollen counts in an epidemiological case-control study [26]. Through increased temperature and concomitant increased CO_2 concentration, plant growth is becoming affected in various ways leading to more, new and altered pollens.

More Pollen

In the last decades a prolonged vegetation period of pollinating plants has been observed in the northern hemisphere with an earlier start of flowering and later foliage, which has led to a prolongation of the pollen season by 10–14 days [16, 17]. Therefore, there is also an increased exposure to outdoor allergens from pollen.

The prolongation of pollination periods has also been shown for birch, which between 1984 and 2008 was approximately 11 days. Independent from pollen counts, there is a variability of allergen content produced by birch pollen as has been shown in various regions in Germany. The clinical relevance of allergen exposure is not totally reflected by pollen counts, but should be measured adequately by allergen content of the ambient air [10].

New Pollen

Through global warming, alterations of fauna and flora have occurred with a shift of vegetation zones of many plants and immigration of neophytes; these are plants which are not classically in the endemic vegetation. In Central Europe more than 800 new plant species and over 1,000 new animal species, especially insects, have been observed over the last 30 years.

In Germany one example of such an allergy-promoting neophyte is *Ambrosia artemisiifolia* (ragweed), a powerful allergen carrier which was extremely rare 30 years ago, but now represents a common aeroallergen in some parts of Germany, especially the Rhine valley, Baden-Württemberg and Southern Bavaria. Sensitization to ragweed can be observed in about 15% of individuals attending an out-patient clinic of the Department of Dermatology and Allergy in Munich. In a prospective study including allergy testing and conjunctival as well as nasal provocation tests, it was found that 30% of ragweed-sensitized individuals are truly allergic, i.e. show a positive provocation test. This means that in Germany, it is very likely that 1–2 million people are already affected by an *Ambrosia* allergy; however, *Ambrosia* is not one of the standard allergens tested in routine allergy practice [7].

Altered Pollen

It has been shown that air pollutants do not only act as irritants on skin and mucus membranes, but – already in the atmosphere – show interactions with allergen carriers such as pollen grains. In the atmosphere over large cities in West Germany, pollen has been found to show agglomeration together with pollutant particles as well as alterations of pollen surface and biological activation of pollen grains.

Pollen has been shown to not only be an allergen carrier, but also to release highly active lipid mediators, such as pollen-associated lipid mediators, which have proinflammatory activity comparable to leukotrienes and immunomodulating effects comparable to prostaglandins [6, 39]. The discovery of these substances might help to explain irritative effects of pollen leading to allergy-like symptoms in individuals who do not suffer from IgE-mediated allergic rhinoconjunctivitis.

Other Allergens

Regarding the effects of climate change on allergy-inducing animals, there is an increased occurrence of caterpillars inducing irritant dermatitis and allergies, namely *Taumatopoea processionaria* (oak processionary caterpillar). It has also been discussed whether the occurrence of hymenoptera, especially wasps (*Vespula vulgaris* or *Vespula germanica*), is increasing during warmer summer periods, giving rise to an increasing incidence of hymenoptera venom anaphylaxis.

Conclusion

There is more and more evidence that environmental factors of various categories can influence the development of allergies. Through increases in the Earth's surface temperature and increased CO_2 concentration in the atmosphere, plant growth may be influenced in such a way that more, new and altered allergens are produced, which in turn can act upon human individuals.

Acknowledgement

This work was supported by the Christine Kühne Center of Allergy Research and Education (CK-CARE).

References

1 Alessandrini F, Schulz H, Takenaka S, et al: Effects of ultrafine carbon particle inhalation on allergic inflammation of the lung. J Allergy Clin Immunol 2006;117:824–230.

2 Asero R: The changing pattern of ragweed allergy in the area of Milan, Italy. Allergy 2007;62:1097–1099.

3 Asher MI, Montefort S, Björksten B, et al: Worldwide time trends in the prevalence of symptoms of asthma, allergic rhinoconjunctivitis, and eczema in childhood: ISAAC Phases One and Three repeat multicountry cross-sectional surveys. Lancet 2006; 368:733–743.

4 Behrendt H: Klimawandel und Allergie; in Gostomzyk JG, Enke M (eds): Globaler Klimawandel und Gesundheit. Munich, Schriftenreihe der Landeszentrale für Gesundheit, 2008, vol 19.

5 Behrendt H, et al: Der Rat vom Sachverständigen für Umweltfragen (SRU). Sondergutachten: Umwelt und Gesundheit. Stuttgart, Metzler-Peschel, 1999.

6 Behrendt H, Becker WM: Localization, release and bioavailability of pollen allergens: the influence of environmental factors. Curr Opin Immunol 2001; 13:709–715.

7 Behrendt H, Gabrio T, Alberternst B, Kaminski U, Nawrath S, Böhme M: Gesundheitliche Bewertung der Verbreitung von Ambrosia artemisiifolia in Baden-Württemberg: Risiko oder Überschätzung? Umweltmed Forsch Prax 2010;15:34–41.

8 Bousquet J, Khaltaev N, Conz AA, et al: Allergic rhinitis and impact on asthma (ARIA) update: in cooperation with World Health Organization WHO, GA2LEN and AllerGEN. Allergy 2008;63:8–160.

9 Braun-Fahrländer C, Gassner M, Grize L, et al: Prevalence of hay fever and allergic sensitization in farmer's children and their peers living in the same rural community. Swiss Study on Childhood Allergy and Respiratory Symptoms with Respect to Air Pollution (SCARPOL). Exp Allergy 1999;29:28–34.

10 Buters JT, Weichenmeier I, Ochs S, Pusch G, Kreyling W, Boere AJ, Schober W, Behrendt H: The allergen Bet v 1 in fractions of ambient air deviates from birch pollen counts. Allergy 2010;65:850–858.
11 Camargo CA Jr, Weiss ST, Zhang S, et al: Prospective study of body mass index, weight change, and risk of adult-onset asthma in women. Arch Intern Med 1999;159:2582–2588.
12 Cookson WO, Moffatt MF: Genetics of asthma and allergic disease. Hum Mol Genet 2000;9:2359–2364.
13 Diaz-Sanchez D, Tsien A, Flemming A, et al: Combined diesel exhaust particulate and ragweed allergen challenge markedly enhances human in vivo ragweed-specific IgE and skews cytokine production to a T helper cell 2-type pattern. J Immunol 1997;158:2406–2413.
14 Ege MJ, Herzum I, Büchele G, et al; Protection against Allergy Study Rural Environments (PASTURE) Study Group: Prenatal exposure to a farm environment modifies atopic sensation at birth. J Allergy Clin Immunol 2008;122:407–412.
15 Eder W, Ege MJ, Von Mutius E: The asthma epidemic. N Engl J Med 2006;355:2226–2235.
16 Estrella N, Menzel A, Krämer U, Behrendt H: Integration of flowering dates in phenology and pollen counts in aerobiology: analysis of their spatial and temporal coherence in Germany (1992–1999). Int J Biometeorol 2006;51:49–59.
17 Fitter AH, Fitter RSR: Rapid change in flowering time in British plants. Science 2002;296:1689–1691.
18 Gassner-Bachmann B, Wüthrich B: Bauernkinder leiden selten an Heuschnupfen und Asthma. Dtsch Med Wschr 2000;125:924–931.
19 Gilliland FD, Li YF, Peters JM: Effects of maternal smoking during pregnancy and environmental tobacco smoke on asthma and wheezing in children. Am J Respir Crit Care Med 2001;163:429–436.
20 Hirsch T, Weiland SK, von Mutius E, et al: Inner city air pollution and respiratory health and atopy in children. Eur Respir J 1999;14:669–677.
21 Holgate ST: Asthma genetics: waiting to exhale. Nat Genet 1997;15:227–229.
22 Confalonieri U, Menne B, Akhtar R, Ebi KL, Hauengue M, Kovats RS, Revich B, Woodward A: Human health; in Parry ML, Canziani OF, Palutikof JP, van der Linden PJ, Hanson CE (eds): Climate Change 2007: Impacts, Adaptation and Vulnerability. Contribution of Working Group II to the Fourth Assessment Report of the Intergovernmental Panel on Climate Change. Cambridge, Cambridge University Press, 2007, pp 391–431.
23 Jörres R, Nowak D, Magnussen H: The effect of ozone exposure on allergen responsiveness in subjects with asthma or rhinitis. Am J Respir Crit Care Med 1996;153:56–64.
24 Kaneko Y, Motohashi Y, Nakamura H, Endo T, Eboshida A: Increasing prevalence of Japanese ceder pollinosis: a meta-regression analysis. Int Arch Allergol Immunol 2005;136:365–371.
25 Koren HS, Bromberg PA: Respiratory responses of asthmatics to ozone. Int Arch Allergy Immunol 1995;107:236–238.
26 Krämer U, Behrendt H, Dolgner R, et al: Airway diseases and allergies in East and West German children during the first 5 years after reunification: time trends and the impact of sulphur dioxide and total suspended particles. Int J Epidemiol 1999;28:865–873.
27 Krämer U, Koch T, Ranft U, et al: Traffic-related air pollution is associated with atopy in children living in urban areas. Epidemiology 2000;11:64–70.
28 Martinez FD, Wright AL, Taussig LM, et al: Asthma and wheezing in the first six years of life. The Group Health Medical Associates. N Engl J Med 1995;332:133–138.
29 Morgenstern V, Zutavern A, Cyrys J, et al: Respiratory health and individual estimated exposure to traffic-related air pollutants in a cohort of young children. Occup Environ Med 2007;64:8–16.
30 Ring J (ed): Epidemiologie allergischer Erkrankungen. Munich, MMW, 1991.
31 Ring J: Allergy and modern society: does 'Western life style' promote the development of allergies? Int Arch Allergy Immunol 1997;113:7–10.
32 Ring J: Allergy in Practice. Berlin, Springer, 2005.
33 Ring J, Bachert C, Bauer C-P, Czech W (eds): Weissbuch Allergie in Deutschland. ed 3. Munich, Urban & Vogel, 2010.
34 Ring J, Krämer U, Schäfer T, Behrendt H: Why are allergies increasing? Curr Opin Immunol 2001;13:701–708.
35 Rogers CA, Wayne PM, Macklin EA, Muilenberg ML, Wagner CJ, Epstein PR, Bazazz FA: Interaction of the onset of spring and elevated atmospheric CO_2 on ragweed (*Ambrosia artemisiifolia* L.) pollen production. Environ Health Perspect 2006;114:865–869.
36 Sporik R, Holgate ST, Platts-Mills TA, et al: Exposure to house-dust mite allergen (Der p I) and the development of asthma in childhood. A prospective study. N Engl J Med 1990;323:502–507.
37 Spengler JD, Samet JM, McCarthy JF (eds): Indoor Air Quality Handbook. New York, McGraw-Hill, 2000.

38 Tang EA, Matsui E, Wiesch DG, Samet JM: Epidemiology of Asthma and Allergic Diseases; in: Middleton's Allergy Principles and Practice, ed 7. St. Loius, Mosby, 2008, pp 1127–1168.
39 Traidl-Hoffmann C, Mariani V, Hochrein H, et al: Pollen-associated phytoprostanes inhibit dendritic cell interleukin-12 production and augment T helper type 2 cell polarization. J Exp Med 2005;201: 627–636.
40 Von Mutius E, Weiland SK, Fritzsch C, et al: Increasing prevalence of hay fever and atopy among children in Leipzig, East Germany. Lancet 1998; 351:862–866.

Prof. Dr. med. Heidrun Behrendt
ZAUM – Zentrum Allergie und Umwelt (Center for Allergy and Environment)
Technische Universität München, Christine Kühne Center for Allergy Research and Education (CK-CARE)
Biedersteiner Strasse 29
DE–80802 Munich (Germany)
Tel. +49 89 4140 3450, Fax +49 89 4140 3452, E-Mail heidrunbehrendt@web.de

Ring J, Darsow U, Behrendt H (eds): New Trends in Allergy and Atopic Eczema.
Chem Immunol Allergy. Basel, Karger, 2012, vol 96, pp 15–23

The Hygiene Hypothesis Does Not Apply to Atopic Eczema in Childhood

Claudia Cramer[a] · Elke Link[a] · Sibylle Koletzko[d] · Irina Lehmann[f] · Joachim Heinrich[c] · H.-Erich Wichmann[c] · Carl-P. Bauer[e] · Andrea v. Berg[b] · Dietrich Berdel[b] · Olf Herbarth[g] · Beate Schaaf[i] · Michael Borte[h] · Heidrun Behrendt[j] · Ursula Krämer[a]

[a]IUF – Leibniz Institut für Umweltmedizinische Forschung an der Heinrich-Heine-Universität, Düsseldorf, [b]Department of Pediatrics, Marien Hospital Wesel, Wesel, [c]Institute of Epidemiology, German Research Center for Environmental Health (GmbH), Helmholtz Zentrum München, Neuherberg, [d]Dr. von Haunersches Kinderspital, Ludwig-Maximilians-Universität, [e]Department of Pediatrics, Technische Universität München and LVA Oberbayern, Munich, [f]Department of Environmental Immunology, UFZ-Centre for Environmental Research, Leipzig, [g]Faculty of Medicine, Environmental Medicine and Environmental Hygiene, University of Leipzig, and [h]Department of Pediatrics, University of Leipzig, Municipal Hospital St. Georg, Leipzig, and [i]Praxis für Kinder- und Jugendmedizin, Bad Honnef, [j]Christine Kühne Center of Allergy Research and Education (CK-CARE), Munich, Germany

Abstract

There is evidence that environmental factors are important for the development of eczema. Different mechanisms have been discussed in the literature, the best known of which is the hygiene hypothesis. However, epidemiological data give reason for questioning this hypothesis with regard to childhood eczema. We present results from two German birth cohort studies (LISAplus and GINIplus) concerning regional prevalence patterns of eczema and the association of eczema with day care center attendance and older siblings. Our findings are not in line with the hygiene hypothesis and question its validity with regard to eczema. It seems reasonable to assume that the effect of environmental factors is somehow disease-specific.

Eczema is the most common inflammatory skin disorder in the pediatric population. In industrialized countries the life-time prevalence of eczema in children ranges from 13 to 37% [1]. Recently, it has been shown that the prevalence of eczema is substantially increasing in many developing countries with formerly low prevalences [2]. There is evidence that environmental factors are important for determining eczema expression [2]. Based on epidemiological studies, different mechanisms have been discussed in order to explain the development of eczema. The best known and most controversial hypothesis is the so-called 'hygiene hypothesis', which was first proposed

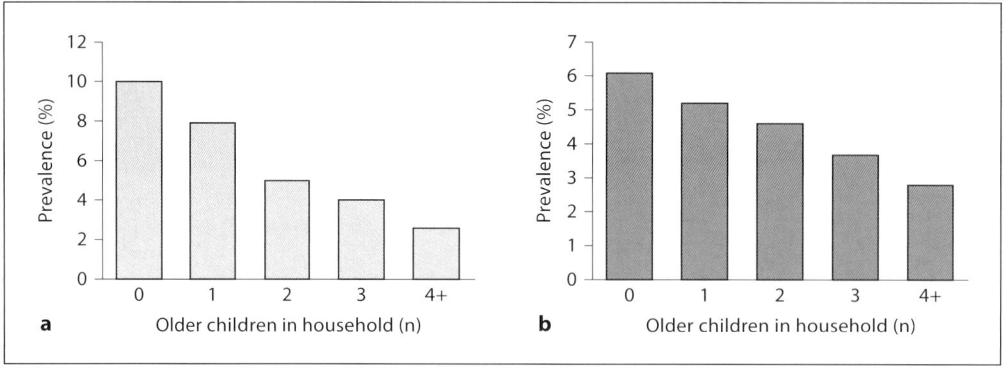

Fig. 1. Prevalence of hay fever in the 11th year of life (**a**) and eczema in the 1st year of life (**b**) by position in the household (adapted from Strachan [3]; National Child Development Study (n = 17,414).

by Strachan [3] in the late 1980s. It is based on the observation that eczema and hay fever is less common in children with larger numbers of older siblings (fig. 1).

Strachan [3] postulated that in industrialized countries, factors like declining family size, improvements in household amenities and higher standards of personal hygiene have led to a lack of exposure to infections in early childhood. This may have resulted in a more widespread clinical expression of atopic diseases in these countries. However, epidemiological data give reason for questioning the hygiene hypothesis [4, 5]. Numerous studies have investigated different environmental exposures related to the hygiene hypothesis, the best known being farming environment [6–8], pet ownership [9–11], Western lifestyle [12], anthroposophic lifestyle [13], older siblings [14, 15] and day care center attendance [16]. Some of our recent results concerning the influence of environmental factors on the development of childhood eczema are presented in the following sections and will be discussed against the background of the hygiene hypothesis.

Eczema in East and West Germany

After the reunification of Germany, several epidemiological studies consistently demonstrated that the prevalence of eczema was higher in children from East Germany than in children from West Germany [12, 17]. In contrast, hay fever and allergic sensitization were significantly less prevalent in East Germany [18]. As shown in figure 2, results from our ongoing birth cohort study LISAplus Influence of Life-style factors on the development of the Immune System and Allergies in East and West Germany Plus (Influence of Life-Style Factors on the Development of the Immune System and Allergies in East and West Germany Plus; n = 3,097) also indicate that prevalence and cumulative incidence up to the age of 6 years are higher in East Germany than in West Germany [19].

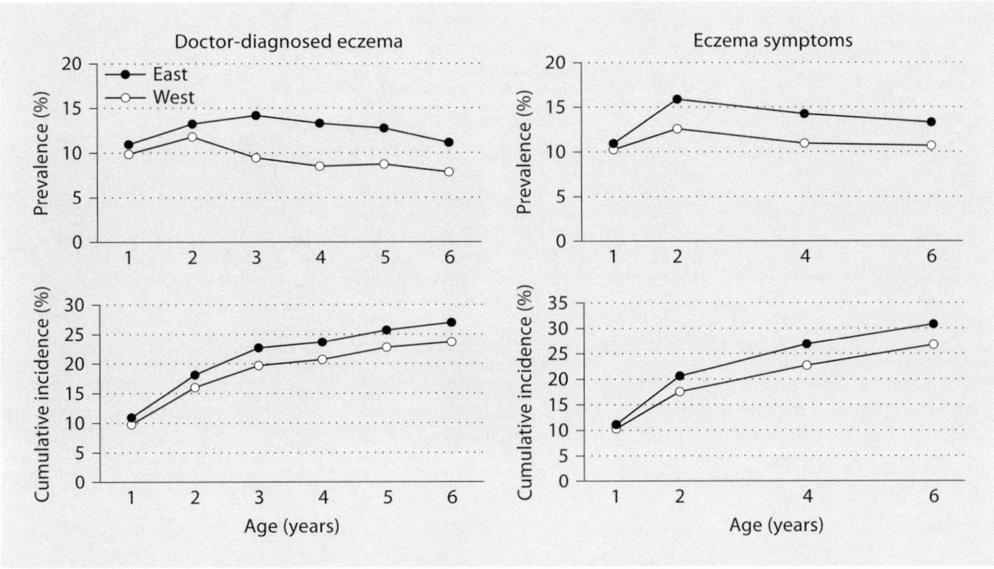

Fig. 2. Prevalence and cumulative incidence of eczema in East and West Germany [19].

Recently, we [20] performed a trend study of 6-year-old children in East and West Germany using data between 1991 and 2000. In accordance with results of other studies [21, 22], we found that the prevalence of hay fever and allergic sensitizations has equalized in East and West Germany, whereas regional differences for eczema still exist: the 1-year prevalence of self-reported eczema symptoms remained stable and the point prevalence of eczema diagnosed by clinical examination decreased in East Germany as well as in West Germany. It has been hypothesized that different regional patterns of allergic diseases are attibutable to factors related to the 'Western lifestyle' [23–26]. However, the causes for the different regional patterns of eczema prevalence in childhood are largely unknown.

Eczema and Day Care Center Attendance

There is a great body of evidence demonstrating that day care attendance is associated with an increased prevalence of respiratory infections early in life [27–30]. According to the hygiene hypothesis, it is postulated that infections during early childhood might protect children from the development of atopic diseases later in life. We [31] showed that in children aged 5–14 years from small families who entered day nursery between the ages of 6 and 11 months, the prevalence of atopic sensitization, asthma and hay fever was lower than in children who entered day nursery at an older age (fig. 3). However, there was no effect of age at entry to day nursery on eczema development.

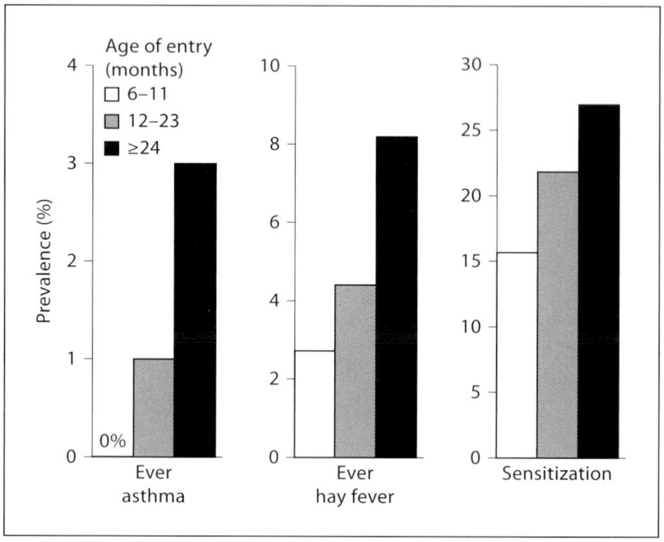

Fig. 3. Doctor-diagnosed allergic diseases and atopy (sensitization against house dust mites or pollen diagnosed by skin prick test) in children from small families (n ≤3) and age of entry to day nursery (Bitterfeld study, n = 663) [31].

In the birth cohort study LISAplus, we investigated different risk factors in East and West Germany that might explain regional differences in eczema prevalence and cumulative incidence [19]. To our knowledge, this is the first longitudinal study that focuses on the identification of explanatory risk factors for regional differences in eczema prevalence between East and West Germany. From a broad range of potential risk factors, we identified day care center attendance in the first 2 years of life as the only explanatory risk factor for the observed regional differences in eczema prevalence and incidence. Early day care center attendance is much more common in East Germany than in West Germany (55.1% in East Germany vs. 5.7% in West Germany). Children, attending day care were at higher risk for eczema regardless of whether they were from East or West Germany (see fig. 4).

We investigated the association between the variable 'East/West' and eczema using the general estimating equation. The OR for the variable 'East/West' was calculated in two different regression models (model before adjusting for day care attendance and model after adjusting for day care attendance; fig. 5).

Before adjusting for day care attendance, the OR for the variable 'East/West' is significantly greater than 1 (OR: 1.48, CI: 1.19–1.85). After additionally adjusting for day care attendance, parameter estimates diminish towards 1 (OR: 1.10, CI: 0.85–1.44). In the adjusted model with day care attendance, the variable 'East/West' is no longer a risk factor for eczema. To the best of our knowledge our study is the first successful attempt to explain East-West differences in the prevalence of atopic diseases based on empirical data. However, these results are in contrast to expectations from the hygiene hypothesis. According to this hypothesis, one might have expected that eczema was less prevalent in children with early day care attendance because children

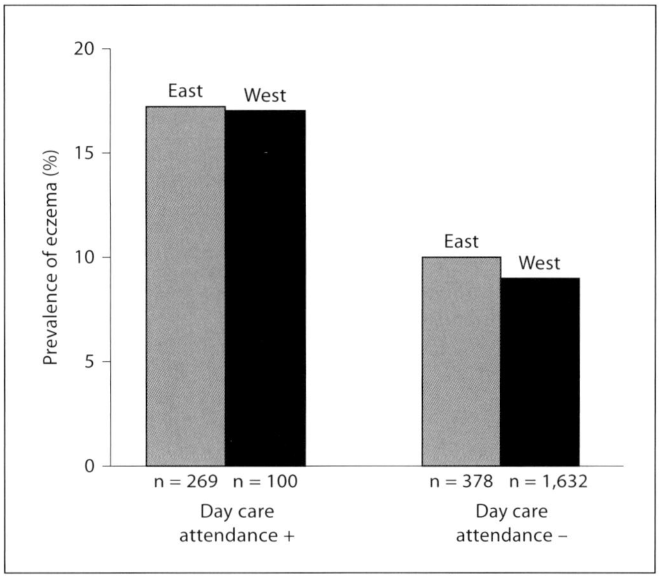

Fig. 4. Prevalence of eczema in children at 3 years of age with and without day care attendance in the birth cohort study LISAplus.

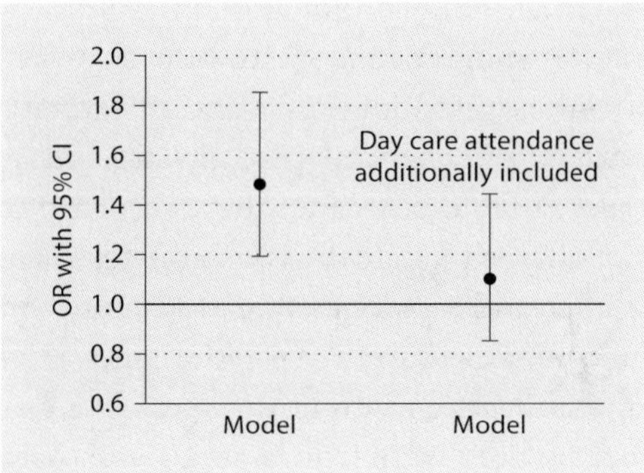

Fig. 5. East-West differences in eczema before and after adjusting for day care center attendance in the birth cohort study LISAplus (n = 2,843). Adjusted for gender and parental allergy.

are seen as a proxy for infections early in life which in turn are assumed to have a protective effect in allergy development.

Eczema, Older Siblings and *FLG* Mutations

Several studies have shown a protective effect of older siblings on eczema development, which is in line with the hygiene hypothesis. However, findings are not consistent [14, 15, 32–35], and there might be different causal pathways for the development of eczema. Barrier disturbances, in particular, as found in children with filaggrin (*FLG*)

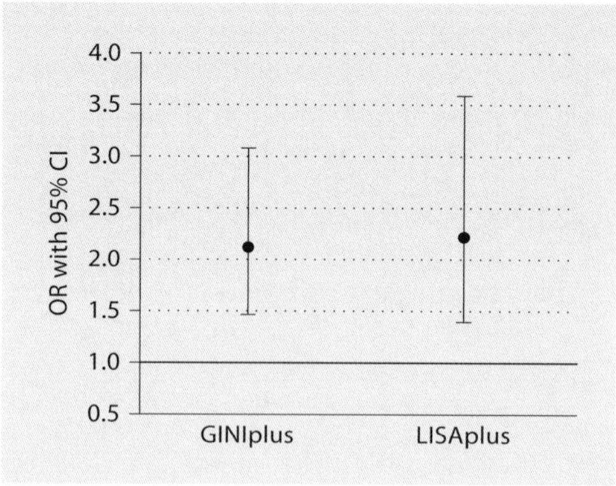

Fig. 6. Association between *FLG* mutations and eczema in the two birth cohort studies GINIplus (n = 1,772) and LISAplus (n = 1,037).

mutations seem to play an important role [36, 37]. We investigated the interaction between *FLG* mutations (R501X, 2282del4) and the presence of older siblings on the development of eczema in the two independent birth cohorts LISAplus (n = 3,097) and GINIplus (German Infant Nutritional Intervention Study Plus Environmental and Genetic Influences on Allergy Development; n = 5,991) [38].

Our results confirm that *FLG* mutations enhance the development of eczema (fig. 6). The risk of developing eczema is more than two times higher in children with mutations than in those without. We found no overall protective effect of older siblings on eczema development. On the contrary, children with *FLG* mutations had a significantly higher risk for eczema if they had older siblings (fig. 7). Attending day care centers lessened this effect. After excluding 303 children who attended early day care, the OR for interaction between *FLG* mutations and older siblings was 3.27 (95% CI: 1.14–9.36) in LISAplus and 2.41 (95% CI: 1.06–5.48) in GINIplus.

Furthermore, we investigated the prevalence of house dust mite sensitization in 6-year-old children stratified for *FLG* mutations and older siblings. As shown in figure 8, the prevalence of sensitization is lower in children with older siblings and without *FLG* mutation as is expected by the hygiene hypothesis. However, children with *FLG* mutations are more often sensitized to house dust mite if they have older siblings. These results are not in line with the hygiene hypothesis.

Instead, they speak in favor of an outside-to-inside pathogenic mechanism in atopic eczema and indicate that skin barrier disturbance may be an important determinant for the effect of microbial or allergen exposures on allergic sensitization. The skin barrier abnormality caused by *FLG* mutations allows an enhanced ingress of allergens, as has recently been shown in mouse models [39, 40]. The presence of older siblings might go along with a higher exposure against allergens and microorganisms. In the case of children with *FLG* loss-of-function mutations having a damaged epithelial barrier, these substances easily penetrate into the subepidermal layer. This might result in a higher predisposition for secondary eczema manifestation and allergic sensitization.

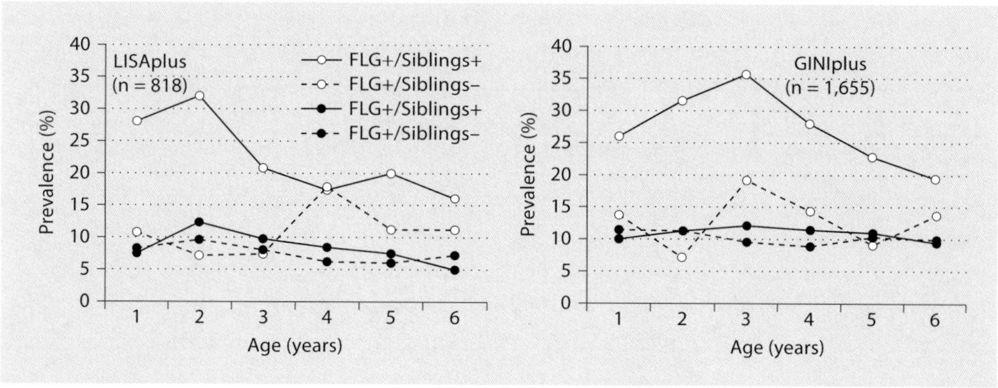

Fig. 7. One-year prevalence of doctor-diagnosed eczema in children up to the age of 6 years stratified for *FLG* mutations and older siblings. Children who attended day care centers in the first 2 years of life were excluded [38].

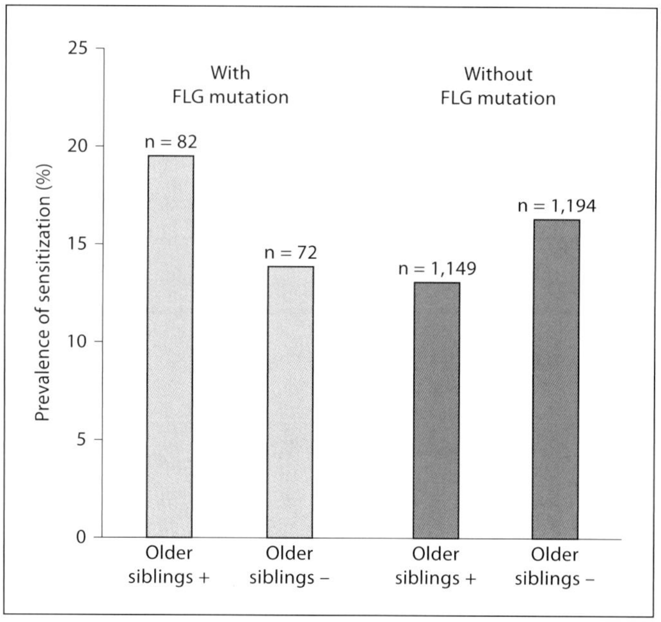

Fig. 8. *FLG* mutations, older siblings and house dust mite sensitization in 6-year-old children in the birth cohort studies LISAplus and GINIplus.

Conclusion

Contrary to the expectations derived from the hygiene hypothesis, we found that eczema is more prevalent in East Germany than in West Germany, more prevalent in children visiting day center attendance during the first 2 years of life, and more prevalent in children with older siblings and *FLG* mutations. Our findings therefore question the validity of the hygiene hypothesis with regard to eczema. It seems reasonable to assume that the effect of environmental factors is somehow disease-specific. There might be a protective effect of day care center attendance or older siblings on the development of hay fever or asthma. However, this does not necessarily apply for eczema. As there are significant differences in the cell organization of the skin and the bronchial or nasal mucosa [41], the relevant risk factors in the onset of the respective atopic disease might also be different.

Acknowledgement

This work was supported by the Christine Kühne Center of Allergy Research and Education (CK-CARE).

References

1 Flohr C, Weinmayr G, Weiland SK, Addo-Yobo E, Annesi-Maesano I, Bjorksten B, et al: How well do questionnaires perform compared with physical examination in detecting flexural eczema? Findings from the International Study of Asthma and Allergies in Childhood (ISAAC) Phase Two. Br J Dermatol 2009;161:846–853.

2 Williams H, Stewart A, von ME, Cookson W, Anderson HR: Is eczema really on the increase worldwide? J Allergy Clin Immunol 2008;121:947–954.

3 Strachan DP: Hay fever, hygiene, and household size. BMJ 1989;299:1259–1260.

4 Matricardi PM: 99th Dahlem Conference on Infection, Inflammation and Chronic Inflammatory Disorders: controversial aspects of the 'hygiene hypothesis'. Clin Exp Immunol 2010;160:98–105.

5 Zutavern A, Hirsch T, Leupold W, Weiland S, Keil U, von Mutius E: Atopic dermatitis, extrinsic atopic dermatitis and the hygiene hypothesis: results from a cross-sectional study. Clin Exp Allergy 2005;35:1301–1308.

6 Braun-Fahrländer C, Lauener R: Farming and protective agents against allergy and asthma. Clin Exp Allergy 2003;33:409–411.

7 Riedler J, Braun-Fahrlander C, Eder W, Schreuer M, Waser M, Maisch S, et al: Exposure to farming in early life and development of asthma and allergy: a cross-sectional survey. Lancet 2001;358:1129–1133.

8 Perkin MR, Strachan DP: Which aspects of the farming lifestyle explain the inverse association with childhood allergy? J Allergy Clin Immunol 2006;117:1374–1381.

9 Chen CM, Morgenstern V, Bischof W, Herbarth O, Borte M, Behrendt H, et al: Dog ownership and contact during childhood and later allergy development. Eur Respir J 2008;31:963–973.

10 Nafstad P, Magnus P, Gaarder PI, Jaakkola JJ: Exposure to pets and atopy-related diseases in the first 4 years of life. Allergy 2001;56:307–312.

11 Ownby DR, Johnson CC, Peterson EL: Exposure to dogs and cats in the first year of life and risk of allergic sensitization at 6 to 7 years of age. JAMA 2002;288:963–972.

12 Schäfer T, Dockery D, Krämer U, Behrendt H, Ring J: Experiences with the severity scoring of atopic dermatitis in a population of German pre-school children. Br J Dermatol 1997;137:558–562.

13 Floistrup H, Swartz J, Bergstrom A, Alm JS, Scheynius A, van Hage M, et al: Allergic disease and sensitization in Steiner school children. J Allergy Clin Immunol 2006;117:59–66.

14 Karmaus W, Botezan C: Does a higher number of siblings protect against the development of allergy and asthma? A review. J Epidemiol Community Health 2002;56:209–217.

15 Benn CS, Melbye M, Wohlfahrt J, Björkstén B, Aaby P: Cohort study of sibling effect, infectious diseases, and risk of atopic dermatitis during first 18 months of life. BMJ 2004;328:1223.

16 Caudri D, Wijga A, Scholtens S, Kerkhof M, Gerritsen J, Ruskamp JM, et al: Early daycare is associated with an increase in airway symptoms in early childhood but is no protection against asthma or atopy at 8 years. Am J Respir Crit Care Med 2009; 180:491–498.

17 Weiland SK, von Mutius E., Hirsch T, Duhme H, Fritzsch C, Werner B, et al: Prevalence of respiratory and atopic disorders among children in the east and west of Germany five years after unification. Eur Respir J 1999;14:862–870.

18 von Mutius E, Martinez FD, Fritzsch C, Nicolai T, Roell G, Thiemann HH: Prevalence of asthma and atopy in two areas of West and East Germany. Am J Respir Crit Care Med 1994;149:358–364.

19 Cramer C, Link E, Bauer CP, Hoffmann U, Von BA, Lehmann I, et al: Association between attendance of day care centres and increased prevalence of eczema in the German birth cohort study LISAplus. Allergy 2011;66:68–75.

20 Krämer U, Oppermann H, Ranft U, Schäfer T, Ring J, Behrendt H: Differences in allergy trends between East and West Germany and possible explanations. Clin Exp Allergy 2010;40:289–298.

21 Brockow I, Zutavern A, Hoffmann U, Grubl A, Von BA, Koletzko S, et al: Early allergic sensitizations and their relevance to atopic diseases in children aged 6 years: results of the GINI study. J Investig Allergol Clin Immunol 2009;19:180–187.

22 Schlaud M, Atzpodien K, Thierfelder W: Allergic diseases. Results from the German Health Interview and Examination Survey for Children and Adolescents (KiGGS) (in German). Bundesgesundheitsblatt Gesundheitsforschung Gesundheitsschutz 2007;50:701–710.

23 Wichmann HE: Possible explanation for the different trends of asthma and allergy in East and West Germany. Clin Exp Allergy 1996;26:621–623.

24 Matricardi PM: Prevalence of atopy and asthma in Eastern versus Western Europe: why the difference? Ann Allergy Asthma Immunol 2001;87:24–27.

25 Heinrich J, Richter K, Magnussen H, Wichmann HE: Is the prevalence of atopic diseases in East and West Germany already converging? Eur J Epidemiol 1998;14:239–245.

26 Vartiainen E, Petays T, Haahtela T, Jousilahti P, Pekkanen J: Allergic diseases, skin prick test responses, and IgE levels in North Karelia, Finland, and the Republic of Karelia, Russia. J Allergy Clin Immunol 2002;109:643–648.

27 Hagerhed-Engman L, Bornehag CG, Sundell J, Aberg N: Day-care attendance and increased risk for respiratory and allergic symptoms in preschool age. Allergy 2006;61:447–453.

28 Buske-Kirschbaum A, Geiben A, Hellhammer D: Psychobiological aspects of atopic dermatitis: an overview. Psychother Psychosom 2001;70:6–16.

29 Zutavern A, Rzehak P, Brockow I, Schaaf B, Bollrath C, Von Berg A, et al: Day care in relation to respiratory-tract and gastrointestinal infections in a German birth cohort study. Acta Paediatr 2007;96: 1494–1499.

30 Celedon JC, Litonjua AA, Weiss ST, Gold DR: Day care attendance in the first year of life and illnesses of the upper and lower respiratory tract in children with a familial history of atopy. Pediatrics 1999;104: 495–500.

31 Krämer U, Heinrich J, Wjst M, Wichmann HE: Age of entry to day nursery and allergy in later childhood. Lancet 1999;353:450–454.

32 Foliaki S, Annesi-Maesano I, Tuuau-Potoi N, Waqatakirewa L, Cheng S, Douwes J, et al: Risk factors for symptoms of childhood asthma, allergic rhinoconjunctivitis and eczema in the Pacific: an ISAAC Phase III study. Int J Tuberc Lung Dis 2008; 12:799–806.

33 Ohfuji S, Miyake Y, Arakawa M, Tanaka K, Sasaki S: Sibship size and prevalence of allergic disorders in Japan: the Ryukyus Child Health Study. Pediatr Allergy Immunol 2009;20:377–384.

34 Harrop J, Chinn S, Verlato G, Olivieri M, Norback D, Wjst M, et al: Eczema, atopy and allergen exposure in adults: a population-based study. Clin Exp Allergy 2007;37:526–535.

35 Purvis DJ, Thompson JM, Clark PM, Robinson E, Black PN, Wild CJ, et al: Risk factors for atopic dermatitis in New Zealand children at 3.5 years of age. Br J Dermatol 2005;152:742–749.

36 Weidinger S, Illig T, Baurecht H, Irvine AD, Rodriguez E, Diaz-Lacava A, et al: Loss-of-function variations within the filaggrin gene predispose for atopic dermatitis with allergic sensitizations. J Allergy Clin Immunol 2006;118:214–219.

37 Palmer CN, Irvine AD, Terron-Kwiatkowski A, Zhao Y, Liao H, Lee SP, et al: Common loss-of-function variants of the epidermal barrier protein filaggrin are a major predisposing factor for atopic dermatitis. Nat Genet 2006;38:441–446.

38 Cramer C, Link E, Horster M, Koletzko S, Bauer CP, Berdel D, et al: Elder siblings enhance the effect of filaggrin mutations on childhood eczema: results from the 2 birth cohort studies LISAplus and GINIplus. J Allergy Clin Immunol 2010;125:1254–1260.

39 Oyoshi MK, Murphy GF, Geha RS: Filaggrin-deficient mice exhibit TH17-dominated skin inflammation and permissiveness to epicutaneous sensitization with protein antigen. J Allergy Clin Immunol 2009;124:485–493, 493.e1.

40 Scharschmidt TC, Man MQ, Hatano Y, Crumrine D, Gunathilake R, Sundberg JP, et al: Filaggrin deficiency confers a paracellular barrier abnormality that reduces inflammatory thresholds to irritants and haptens. J Allergy Clin Immunol 2009;124:496–506, 506.e1–6.

41 Akdis M: The cellular orchestra in skin allergy; are differences to lung and nose relevant? Curr Opin Allergy Clin Immunol 2010;10:443–451.

Dr. Claudia Cramer
IUF – Leibniz-Institut für Umweltmedizinische Forschung an der Heinrich-Heine-Universität
Auf'm Hennekamp 50
DE–40225 Düsseldorf (Germany)
Tel. +49 211 3389 284, E-Mail Claudia.cramer@uni-duesseldorf.de

Ring J, Darsow U, Behrendt H (eds): New Trends in Allergy and Atopic Eczema.
Chem Immunol Allergy. Basel, Karger, 2012, vol 96, pp 24–29

Molecular Genetics of Atopic Eczema

Johannes Ring[a] · Matthias Möhrenschlager[c] · Stephan Weidinger[b]

[a]Department of Dermatology and Allergy Biederstein, Technische Universität München, Munich, and [b]Department Dermatology and Allergology, University of Kiel, Kiel, Germany; [c]Hochgebirgsklinik Davos, Davos, Switzerland

Abstract

In both clinical experience and molecular genetic studies, atopic diseases (asthma, rhinoconjunctivitis and eczema) have been found to be strongly genetically influenced. The epidermal protein filaggrin seems to play a crucial role and is encoded within the so-called epidermal differentiation complex on chromosome 1. Filaggrin mutations predispose significantly to an increased risk to develop atopic eczema. Apart from filaggrin, other proteins involved in skin barrier functions such as lipid synthesis and metabolism, protease or protease inhibitor functions also seem to play a role. Besides skin barrier function, immune deviation versus a Th2 dominance and increased IgE production is also genetically determined. Polymorphisms have been found in genes encoding IL-4, IL-13 and STAT-6, and recently a polymorphism on the high-affinity IgE receptor gene has been found. Using genome-wide association studies, new genes with yet unknown functions have been determined to be associated with atopy and atopic eczema.

It has been known for a long time that the classical atopic diseases, namely bronchial asthma, allergic rhinoconjunctivitis and atopic eczema, run within families and show a genetic predisposition [1–3]. Because of this observation, Coca and Cooke [4] came up with the new term 'atopy' in order to better describe this phenomenon. While in childhood, eczema is the most prominent manifestation of atopy, it is allergic rhinoconjunctivitis (commonly called 'hay fever') in adults.

With regard to occurrence throughout one's lifetime, it is most often atopic eczema which is the first manifestation in the first 2 years of life, followed by asthma, while allergic rhinitis develops more slowly in adolescence and reaches its maximum in young adults. Atopic diseases can occur at the same time or in alternating phases of life, a phenomenon which has been called the 'allergic march' or the 'change of floors' ('Etagenwechsel') [1].

Classical Genetics

It has been shown that many patients suffering from atopic eczema also suffer from other atopic diseases in their personal or family history. Approximately 70–80% of the patients with atopic eczema also suffer from airway atopic disease at least once during their lifetime [1, 2].

The use of twin studies is the classical method of proving genetic susceptibility for a certain disease. Monozygotic twins were found to suffer much more often from atopic eczema (about 80%) compared to dizygotic twins who only showed a prevalence of about 20% [5]. Thus, atopic diseases are similar to Crohn's disease or type I diabetes, which also are strongly genetically influenced.

Uehara in Japan was the first to stress the importance of 'descendant' family history in atopic eczema; compared to ascendant family history, where some information may not be remembered, the descendant family history seems to be more reliable for investigation. In 270 families where either the father or mother suffered from atopic eczema, 316 out of 529 children (60%) suffered from atopic eczema. When only one parent was suffering from atopic eczema, the prevalence was 59%; however, when both parents had atopic eczema, 81% of the children were affected by eczema [1].

Linkage Studies

The traditional way to associate a certain clinical marker ('phenotype') to a genetic locus is a segregation study and the calculation of the LOD score (log of the odds). In linkage studies, it has been shown that strong associations can be found for atopic eczema on many chromosomes, but also for asthma or psoriasis. Surprisingly, in some studies there seems to be greater overlap between eczema and psoriasis than between eczema and asthma [6].

Genes of Skin Barrier Function

Using the candidate gene approach, the most exciting progress came from studying the genes for the epidermal protein filaggrin within the so-called epidermal differentiation complex on chromosome 1. In this region a variety of S100 proteins, as well as hornerin and loricrin, are encoded.

Filaggrin was found to be a decisive gene which is absent or reduced in function in the autosomal dominant disease ichthyosis vulgaris, but in a heterozygous way, loss-of-function mutations were found to be a major predisposing factor for the development of atopic eczema [7–9].

Filaggrin is a protein derived from the precursor profilaggrin, which is stored in the keratohyalin granules in the stratum granulosum of the epidermis and formed by dephosphorylation and protein cleavage. The function of filaggrin is to aggregate the keratin filaments in the stratum corneum to form the cornified cell envelope, which then together with epidermal lipids represents the physicochemical basis of the epidermal skin barrier function. Finally, filaggrin is further broken down by proteases to amino acids that contribute to the hygroscopic milieu and acidic pH, and may also have immunomodulatory effects via urocanic acid [10, 11, 41].

Many authors have found a significant association between filaggrin mutation and the risk to develop atopic eczema [12–16]. In another meta-analysis, Rodriguez et al. [15] showed that the filaggrin polymorphism represents a robust risk factor for atopic eczema with a prevalence of 7.5% FLG mutations in controls, while affected individuals show a rate of 21.7%. Therefore, the increased risk to develop atopic eczema in filaggrin mutation carriers can be calculated as having an OR of 3.12.

Functional studies have shown that filaggrin carriers have a significantly reduced natural moisturizing factor concentration in the epidermis compared to healthy non-carriers [11].

Some of the so-called atopy stigmata have also been found to be associated with the filaggrin mutation, especially palmoplantar hyperlinearity (ichthyotic palms) and xerosis (dry skin).

For some time it was questioned whether filaggrin mutations also predispose to asthma; filaggrin mutations are no risk factor for asthma per se, except for the occurrence of eczema plus asthma in one individual [14, 15].

Apart from filaggrin, there are other proteins involved in the skin barrier function, such as in lipid synthesis and metabolism or in protease or protease inhibitor function (e.g. Netherton syndrome).

Genes Involved in IgE-Mediated Hypersensitivity

Atopic diseases are strongly associated with increased IgE synthesis [2, 17–22]. Associations have been found to polymorphisms in genes for IL-4 as well as IL-13 [23, 24]. Equally, polymorphisms in the IgE-relevant signal transduction molecule STAT6 have been found to be associated with circulating IgE levels [25]. Additionally, an association between IgE production and polymorphisms on several molecules of the high-affinity IgE receptor FcERI has been found [26]. Furthermore, gene variants within the innate immune system cascade have been found to be associated with atopic eczema, e.g. regarding the signal transduction molecules NOD1, CARD4 and the Toll-like receptor 9 promoter [27–29].

In a genome-wide association study using serum total IgE as a readout, it was found that a promoter polymorphism on the gene for the high-affinity IgE receptor was strongly associated with IgE levels in serum and specific IgE-mediated sensitization. There was no association with the diseases eczema or asthma per se; however, there was a weak association with the extrinsic ('atopic') variants of atopic eczema and asthma [26, 30–37].

Another association was found with a gene on chromosome 5 involved in DNA repair on a conserved region with a nonregulatory function on the Th2 cytokine transcription (RAD 50). This locus is strongly epigenetically regulated and there is a hypothesis that polymorphisms on this gene might influence DNA methylation [38].

Genes with Unknown Function

In the first genome-wide association study using manifest atopic eczema as a readout, it was found that a common variant on chromosome 11q13 is associated with atopic eczema [39]. The function of this novel gene locus with regard to the pathophysiology of atopic eczema has remained unexplained. A protein encoded on chromosome 11q13 has also been identified as a susceptibility gene for Crohn's disease and is involved in chromatin remodeling, DNA repair and transcription regulation. However, its role in cutaneous inflammation is unclear. The significant association for this 11q13 locus has been replicated independently by another study [40]. In the same genome-wide association study, another risk gene for atopic eczema was identified within the epidermal differentiation complex, independently from the already known filaggrin mutation and possibly associated with the epidermal protein hornerin.

Conclusions

Atopic diseases (asthma, rhinoconjunctivitis and eczema) have been found to be strongly genetically influenced both in clinical experience and in molecular genetic studies. This genetic predisposition does not only affect the immune reactivity in the sense of an immune deviation versus Th2 dominance and IgE production, but also the integrity of the epidermal barrier function.

Acknowledgement

This work was supported by the Christine Kühne Center of Allergy Research and Education (CK-CARE).

References

1 Ring J, Przybilla B, Ruzicka T (eds): Handbook of Atopic Eczema, ed 2. Berlin, Springer, 2006.

2 Wüthrich B: Neurodermitis atopica sive constitutionalis. Ein pathogenetisches Modell aus der Sicht des Allergologen. Aktuel Dermatol 1983;9:1–7.

3 Wüthrich B, Schmid-Grendelmeier P: The atopic eczema/dermatitis syndrome. Epidemiology, natural course, and immunology of the IgE-associated ('extrinsic') and the nonallergic ('intrinsic') AEDS. J Investig Allergol Clin Immunol 2003;13:1–5.

4 Coca A, Cooke R: On the classification of the phenomena of hypersensitiveness. J Immunol 1923;8: 163–182.

5 Schultz Larsen F: Atopic dermatitis: a genetic-epidemiologic study in a population-based twin sample. J Am Acad Dermatol 1993;28:719–723.

6 Cookson WO, Young RP, et al: Maternal inheritance of atopic IgE responsiveness on chromosome 11q. Lancet 1992;340:381–384.

7 Palmer CN, Irvine AD, et al: Common loss-of-function variants of the epidermal barrier protein filaggrin are a major predisposing factor for atopic dermatitis. Nat Genet 2006;38:441–446.

8 Sandilands A, Terron-Kwiatkowski A, et al: Comprehensive analysis of the gene encoding filaggrin uncovers prevalent and rare mutations in ichthyosis vulgaris and atopic eczema. Nat Genet 2007; 39:650–654.

9 Smith FJ, Irvine AD, et al: Loss-of-function mutations in the gene encoding filaggrin cause ichthyosis vulgaris. Nat Genet 2006;38:337–342.

10 Jungersted JM, Scheer H, et al: Stratum corneum lipids, skin barrier function and filaggrin mutations in patients with atopic eczema. Allergy 2010;65:911–918.

11 Kezic S, O'Regan GM, et al: Levels of filaggrin degradation products are influenced by both filaggrin genotype and atopic dermatitis severity. Allergy 2011;66:934–940.

12 Weidinger S, Illig T, et al: Loss-of-function variations within the filaggrin gene predispose for atopic dermatitis with allergic sensitizations. J Allergy Clin Immunol 2006;118:214–219.

13 Baurecht H, Irvine AD, et al: Toward a major risk factor for atopic eczema: meta-analysis of filaggrin polymorphism data. J Allergy Clin Immunol 2007; 120:1406–1412.

14 Rodriguez E, Baurecht H, et al: Meta-analysis of filaggrin polymorphisms in eczema and asthma: robust risk factors in atopic disease. J Allergy Clin Immunol 2009;123:1361–1370.e7.

15 Rodriguez E, Illig T, et al: Filaggrin loss-of-function mutations and association with allergic diseases. Pharmacogenomics 2008;9:399–413.

16 Weidinger S, Rodriguez E, et al: Filaggrin mutations strongly predispose to early-onset and extrinsic atopic dermatitis. J Invest Dermatol 2007;127:724–726.

17 Bieber T, de la Salle H, et al: Human epidermal Langerhans cells express the high affinity receptor for immunoglobulin E (Fc epsilon RI). J Exp Med 1992;175:1285–1290.

18 Bruijnzeel-Koomen CA, van Wichen DF, Spry CJ, Venge P, Bruynzeel PL: Active participation of eosinophils in the patch test reactions to inhalant allergens in atopic dermatitis. Br J Dermatol 1988; 18:229–238.

19 Darsow U, Vieluf D, Ring J: The atopy patch test: an increased rate of reactivity in patients who have an air-exposed pattern of eczema. Br J Dermatol 1996; 135:182–186.

20 Darsow U, Vieluf D, et al: Evaluating the relevance of aeroallergen sensitization in atopic eczema with the atopy patch test: a randomized, double-blind multicenter study. Atopy Patch Test Study Group. J Am Acad Dermatol 1999;40:187–193.

21 Johansson SG, Bieber T, et al: Revised nomenclature for allergy for global use: report of the Nomenclature Review Committee of the World Allergy Organization, October 2003. J Allergy Clin Immunol 2004; 113:832–836.

22 Ring J: Allergy in Practice. Berlin, Springer, 2005.

23 Kawashima T, Noguchi E, et al: Linkage and association of an interleukin 4 gene polymorphism with atopic dermatitis in Japanese families. J Med Genet 1998;35:502–504.

24 Novak N, Kruse S, et al: Dichotomic nature of atopic dermatitis reflected by combined analysis of monocyte immunophenotyping and single nucleotide polymorphisms of the interleukin-4/interleukin-13 receptor gene: the dichotomy of extrinsic and intrinsic atopic dermatitis. J Invest Dermatol 2002;119: 870–875.

25 Weidinger S, Klopp N, et al: Association of a STAT 6 haplotype with elevated serum IgE levels in a population based cohort of white adults. J Med Genet 2004;41:658–663.

26 Weidinger S, Gieger C, et al: Genome-wide scan on total serum IgE levels identifies FCER1A as novel susceptibility locus. PLoS Genet 2008;4:1–9.

27 Novak N, Yu CF, et al: Putative association of a TLR9 promoter polymorphism with atopic eczema. Allergy 2007;62:766–772.

28 Weidinger S, Klopp N, et al: Association of CARD15 polymorphisms with atopy-related traits in a population-based cohort of Caucasian adults. Clin Exp Allergy 2005;35:866–872.
29 Weidinger S, Klopp N, et al: Association of NOD1 polymorphisms with atopic eczema and related phenotypes. J Allergy Clin Immunol 2005;116:177–184.
30 Liu X, Nickel R, et al: An IL13 coding region variant is associated with a high total serum IgE level and atopic dermatitis in the German multicenter atopy study (MAS-90). J Allergy Clin Immunol 2000;106: 167–170.
31 Chen CM, Weidinger S, et al: Common variants in FCER1A influence total serum IgE levels from cord blood up to six years of life. Allergy 2009; 64:1327–1332.
32 Fields PE, Lee GR, et al: Th2-specific chromatin remodeling and enhancer activity in the Th2 cytokine locus control region. Immunity 2004;21: 865–876.
33 Henderson J, Northstone K, et al: 'The burden of disease associated with filaggrin mutations: a population-based, longitudinal birth cohort study.' J Allergy Clin Immunol 2008;121:872–877 e879.
34 Koh BH, Hwang SS, et al: Th2 LCR is essential for regulation of Th2 cytokine genes and for pathogenesis of allergic asthma. Proc Natl Acad Sci USA 2010;107:10614–10619.
35 Lee GR, Fields PE, et al: Regulation of the Th2 cytokine locus by a locus control region. Immunity 2003;19:145–153.
36 Lee GR, Spilianakis CG, et al: Hypersensitive site 7 of the TH2 locus control region is essential for expressing TH2 cytokine genes and for long-range intrachromosomal interactions. Nat Immunol 2005; 6:42–48.
37 Marsh DG, Neely JD, Breazeale DR, Ghosh B, Freidhoff LR, et al: Linkage analysis of IL4and other chromosome 5q31.1 markers and total serum immunoglobulin E concentracions. Science 1994; 264:1152–1156.
38 Li X, Howard TD, et al: Genome-wide association study of asthma identifies RAD50-IL13 and HLA-DR/DQ regions. J Allergy Clin Immunol 2010;125: 328–335 e311.
39 Esparza-Gordillo J, Weidinger S, et al: A common variant on chromosome 11q13 is associated with atopic dermatitis. Nat Genet 2009;41:596–601.
40 O'Regan GM, Campbell LE, et al: Chromosome 11q13.5 variant associated with childhood eczema: an effect supplementary to filaggrin mutations. J Allergy Clin Immunol 2010;125:170–174, e171–172.
41 Mildner M, Jin J, et al: Knockdown of filaggrin impairs diffusion barrier function and increases UV sensitivity in a human skin model. J Invest Dermatol 2010;130:2286–2294.

Prof. Dr. med. Dr. phil. Johannes Ring
Klinik und Poliklinik für Dermatologie und Allergologie Biederstein, Technische Universität München
Christine Kühne Center of Allergy Research and Education (CK-CARE)
Biedersteiner Strasse 29
DE–80802 Munich (Germany)
Tel. +49 89 4140 3170, E-Mail johannes.ring@lrz.tum.de

Ring J, Darsow U, Behrendt H (eds): New Trends in Allergy and Atopic Eczema.
Chem Immunol Allergy. Basel, Karger, 2012, vol 96, pp 30–38

Mechanisms of Immune Tolerance to Allergens

Hiroyuki Fujita[a,b,c] · Norbert Meyer[a] · Mübeccel Akdis[a] · Cezmi A. Akdis[a]

[a]Swiss Institute of Allergy and Asthma Research (SIAF), University of Zurich, Davos, [b]Christine Kühne Center for Allergy Research and Education (CK-CARE), Davos, Switzerland , and [c]Department of Environmental Immuno-Dermatology, Yokohama City University Graduate School of Medicine, Yokohama, Japan

Abstract

In allergic diseases, immune responses are induced by normally well-tolerated allergens, which result in chronic inflammation characterized by antibody secretion and T cell activation. For almost 100 years, allergen-specific immunotherapy (allergen-SIT) has been the potentially curative and antigen-specific method for the treatment of allergic diseases. Allergen-SIT alters the course of allergic diseases and can reduce allergic symptoms and medication use. The key mechanism behind allergen-SIT is the induction of peripheral T cell tolerance by altering the balance between Th cells and regulatory T cells. Both naturally occurring thymus-derived FOXP3$^+$CD4$^+$CD25$^+$ regulatory T cells and inducible type 1 regulatory T cells suppress the development of allergic diseases via several mechanisms including suppression of dendritic cells, Th cells, mast cells, eosinophils and basophils; suppression of inflammatory cell migration to tissues; and decrease of the ratio between allergen-specific IgE and IgG4 antibodies. These effects are mainly mediated by the suppressive cytokines IL-10 and TGF-β. Knowledge of this molecular basis is crucial to understanding the regulation of the immune response and their possible therapeutic applications for allergic diseases.

The immune system has the capacity to protect the host from a number of pathogens while keeping a state of tolerance to self- and innocuous non-self-antigens. Allergies arise as a direct consequence of dysregulated immune responses when immune tolerance to normally harmless antigens is not established. Allergen-specific immunotherapy (allergen-SIT) by the administration of increasing doses of allergen extracts remains the single curative treatment of allergic diseases. Allergen-SIT modifies the course of the disease by establishing long-term tolerance against allergens and restoring the immune balance [1, 2]. The aim of this review is to discuss the mechanisms of allergen-SIT and the current approaches in research and clinical use of allergen-specific immune tolerance induction in allergic diseases.

Pathogenesis of Allergic Diseases

The immune mechanisms underlying allergic diseases can be divided into the sensitization and memory phase, and the effector phase. During the sensitization phase, the differentiation and clonal expansion of allergen-specific $CD4^+$ Th2 cells, which produce IL-4 and IL-13, are essential to induce class switching to the ε-immunoglobulin heavy chain in B cells and the production of allergen-specific IgE antibodies. Allergen-specific IgE binds to the high-affinity receptor of IgE, the FcεRI, on the surface of mast cells and basophils. This activation leads to the sensitization of the patients against a specific allergen [3]. The effector phase is initiated when the patients are re-exposed to the sensitized allergen. The receptor-bound IgE molecule is activated and mediators are released that lead to the development of type I hypersensitivity reaction [4]. During the effector phase, IL-4, IL-5, IL-9 and IL-13 secreted by Th2 cells increase eosinophilia, mucus production and recruitment of inflammatory cells to inflamed tissues. In addition, $CD4^+$ naive T cells also differentiate into distinct T cell subsets such as Th1-, Th9-, Th17- and Th22-type memory and effector cells depending on the status of the cells and existing cytokines in the microenvironment [5]. Th1 cells secrete IFN-γ and induce apoptosis of the epithelial cells and/or smooth muscle cells in patients with asthma and of the keratinocytes in patients with atopic dermatitis [6, 7]. Th1 also induce IL-32, which is detected in chronic skin lesions from patients with atopic dermatitis and increases keratinocyte apoptosis, suggesting that IL-32 plays a role in eczema formation [8]. Apoptosis of activated tissue cells is an important process to limit immune reactions because it eliminates tissue cells secreting chemokines and cytokines, and can therefore break the amplification of inflammatory reactions. In patients with atopic disorders, increased tendency to activation-induced cell death of high IFN-γ-producing Th1 cells is commonly observed leading to Th2 predominance [9]. Recently, IL-25 and IL-33 were discovered as potent inducers of Th2 immunity. IL-33 is released by apoptotic or necrotic tissue cells and IL-25 is mainly secreted by Th2 cells, eosinophils, basophils and mast cells. Both cytokines, IL-25 and IL-33, enhance the secretion of IL-5 and IL-13 by Th2 cells and Th2-type inflammation in the lung or gut [5].

The fundamental role of regulatory T cells to suppress immune response has been shown in many diseases including allergy, asthma, autoimmune diseases and allograft rejection by restoring immune tolerance to allergens, self-antigens or alloantigens. In allergic diseases, regulatory T cells suppress Th2 immune response, dendritic cells (DCs), mast cells, basophils, eosinophils and allergen-specific IgE production and increase of IgG4 and IgA production. They are classified in naturally occurring, thymic selected $FOXP3^+CD4^+CD25^+$ regulatory T cells and inducible regulatory T cells with, in principle, the same surface markers. In addition, T regulatory type 1 (Tr1) cells are generated in the periphery under tolerogenic conditions which secrete IL-10 and TGF-β, but do not express FOXP3. Tr1 cells play a key role in allergen tolerance and they can be induced by allergen-SIT in humans [10, 11]. FOXP3 acts as master switch transcription factor for development and function of thymic selected regulatory T cells [12]. FOXP3 mutations in humans lead to the X-linked immune dysregulation polyendocrinopathy enteropathy syndrome. Patients with this syndrome represent allergic and autoimmune phenotypes due to mutations in FOXP3 leading to nonfunctional regulatory T cells. Recently, it has been demonstrated that FOXP3 directly interacts with the Runt-related transcription factor 1 (RUNX1), which reduces IL-2 and IFN-γ expressions and exerts suppressive functions [13]. Moreover, a novel molecular mechanism associated with TGF-β and FOXP3 expression in humans has been demonstrated [14]. The induction of RUNX1 and RUNX3 by TGF-β plays a critical role in the generation and suppressive functions of induced regulatory T cells. Both RUNX1 and RUNX3 bind to the FOXP3 promoter region and activate the induction of regulatory T cells with the functional expression of FOXP3.

Although the main suppressive cytokines secreted by regulatory T cells are IL-10 and TGF-β, several novel suppressive cytokines have been described recently. IL-35 is constitutively secreted by FOXP3$^+$ regulatory T cells and induces IL-10 production from CD4$^+$CD25$^+$ regulatory T cells increasing their regulatory capacity and IFN-γ production in CD4$^+$CD25$^-$ effector T cells [15, 16]. Therefore, IL-35 might increase the ratio between regulatory T and Th2 cells as well as the ratio between Th1 and Th2 cells, indicating that IL-35 is important for restoring the disturbed immune balance in allergic diseases. In addition, it was recently shown that naive T cells differentiated in the presence of IL-35 to a novel regulatory T cell subset, which mediates suppression via IL-35, but not via IL-10 or TGF-β [17]. The immune regulatory capacity of IL-35 was also demonstrated by the improvement of collagen-induced arthritis in mice after IL-35 treatment [16].

Apart from thymic selected regulatory T cells and inducible regulatory T cells, several other T cells with regulatory functions have been demonstrated. CD8+CD28– T cells have suppressor capacities in vitro sufficient to prevent upregulation of B7 molecules induced by helper T cells on professional antigen-presenting cells, which is an important mechanism for the development of oral tolerance [18]. TCRαβ$^+$CD4$^-$CD8$^-$ double-negative regulatory T cells have been shown to suppress antigen-specific immune responses mediated by CD4$^+$ T and CD8$^+$ T cells in humans and mice [19]. Moreover, natural killer cells have the capacity to suppress antigen-specific T cell response [20]. A certain subset of invariant natural killer T cells also has suppressive functions. The combination of IL-27 and IFN-γ produced by invariant natural killer T cells suppresses established Th2 functions in mice [21]. Antigen-containing liposomal α-galactosylceramide, which is a representative ligand for invariant natural killer T cells, suppresses antigen-specific IgE via induction of tolerogenic DCs and regulatory T cells [22].

B Regulatory Cells

Recently, research has focused on the regulatory function of B cells. B cells produce and secrete antibodies. Thus, B cells are the central cellular component of humoral immune responses. In addition, B cells can modulate CD4$^+$ T cell responses by presenting antigens, stimulating with costimulatory molecules or producing cytokines

[23]. Besides secreting proinflammatory cytokines, B cells are also a dominant source of IL-10. Regulatory B cells regulate the development, proliferation and maintenance of $CD4^+$ T effector cells, memory T cells and regulatory T cells via IL-10 secretion. Several phenotypically distinct populations of IL-10-producing regulatory B cells exist. Transitional 2-marginal zone precursor B cells expressing $CD1d^{hi}CD21^{hi}CD23^+IgM^+$, follicular B cells and B cells expressing high levels of CD1d can produce IL-10 [24]. Transfer of $CD1d^{hi}CD5^+CD19^{hi}$ regulatory B cells prevents the $CD4^+$ T cell-dependent contact hypersensitivity in mice [25]. Since this suppressive function is antigen dependent, regulatory B cells from mice primed with an antigen were not able to suppress the T cell inflammation primed with another antigen. In addition, $CD24^{hi}CD27^+$ B cells can negatively regulate monocyte cytokine production via IL-10-dependent pathways [26]. Taken together, antigen-specific regulatory B cells can sufficiently suppress immune reactions and are potent candidates for the induction of tolerance in allergies. Their function during allergen-specific immunotherapy is not yet known and should be investigated in the future.

Mechanisms of Allergen-Specific Immunotherapy

Role of T Cells

The aim of allergen-SIT is to induce peripheral T cell tolerance, modulate the thresholds for mast cell and basophil activation, and decrease IgE-mediated histamine release [1]. Peripheral T cell tolerance is characterized by generation of allergen-specific Tr1 type regulatory T cells, which produce anti-inflammatory cytokines such as IL-10 and TGF-β. Several studies have demonstrated that allergen-specific Tr1 cells are predominant in healthy individuals to prevent unwanted immune response to nonpathogenic environmental antigens, which lead to allergy [27, 28].

There are two human models showing high-dose exposure to the offending allergens leads to tolerance induction. One is venom allergen and the other is cat allergen. During the beekeeping season, beekeepers are highly exposed to bee venom allergens. Repeated exposure of venom allergens results in a reduction in T cell-related cutaneous late-phase reactions and impaired capacity of allergen-specific T cells to proliferate and produce Th1 and Th2 cytokines. It leads to suppression of allergen-specific unfavorable immune response by Th1 and Th2 cells and this response persists as long as venom exposure is continuous, but returns to the initial level within several months after the end of the beekeeping season. This phenomenon correlates with a clonal switch of venom antigen-specific Th1 and Th2 cells toward IL-10-secreting Tr1 cells. In this model, histamine receptor 2 is upregulated on specific Th2 cells and plays bilateral roles in the suppression of allergen-stimulated T cells and the induction of IL-10 production [29]. It is supported by the findings that the ratio of allergen-specific IgG4 to allergen-specific IgE is much higher in nonallergic beekeepers compared with that in individuals allergic to bee venom. The other high-dose allergen exposure model

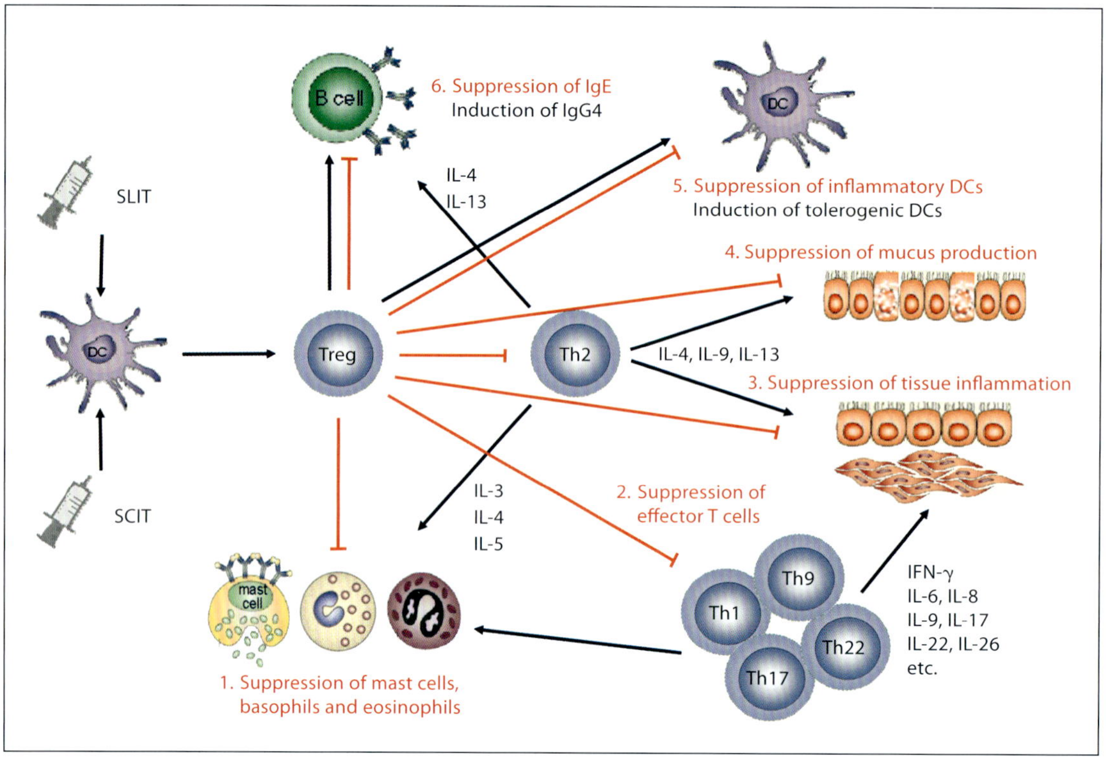

Fig. 1. Mechanisms of allergen-specific immunotherapy and the role of regulatory T cells in allergic diseases. During allergen-SIT, an allergen is internalized by DCs, presented to T cells and antigen-specific naive T cells are polarized. Regulatory T cells suppress the excess allergic responses directly and indirectly by the following mechanisms: (1) suppression of mast cells, basophils and eosinophils; (2) suppression of effector T cells; (3) suppression of inflammatory cell migration to tissues and tissue inflammation; (4) suppression of inflammatory DCs and induction of tolerogenic DCs; and (5) suppression of allergen-specific IgE and induction of IgG4 from B cells. SCIT = Subcutaneous immunotherapy; Treg = regulatory T cell.

with cat allergens also demonstrated the increase of allergen-specific IgG4 and IL-10-producing Tr1 cells without subsequent development of new sensitizations [30].

Role of Allergen-Specific IgG4

IgG4 is thought to capture the allergen before reaching the effector cell-bound IgE, thus preventing the activation of mast cells and basophils [1]. IgG4 antibodies can be used as a marker of introduced allergen dose, and they have the ability to modulate the immune response to allergen. Allergen-specific IgG might be directed against the same epitopes as IgE, resulting in direct competition for allergen binding and a blocking effect. Allergen-SIT also influences the blocking activity on IgE-mediated responses by IgG4. Successful allergen-SIT is associated with an increase in IgG-blocking activity that is not solely dependent on the quantity of IgG antibodies [1]. It seems to be relevant to measure the blocking activity, affinity, or both, of allergen-specific IgG or IgG subsets such as IgG4 and IgG1 instead of their levels in sera. Allergen-SIT induces a transient increase of specific IgE levels in serum, followed by a gradual decrease over months or years of treatment. Serum IgE levels cannot explain the diminished responsiveness to specific allergens because the decrease of serum IgE levels is relatively late and not correlated with clinical improvement after SIT. The decrease in IgE/IgG4 ratio during allergen-SIT is a feature of skewing from allergen-specific Th2 to regulatory T cell predominance. IL-10 is a potent suppressor of total and allergen-specific IgE, whereas it simultaneously increases IgG4 production [31]. Thus IL-10 not only generates tolerance in T cells, but also regulates specific isotype formation toward a noninflammatory phenotype.

Regulation of Basophils, Eosinophils and Mast Cells

Allergen-SIT efficiently modulates the thresholds for mast cell, eosinophil and basophil activation and decreases IgE-mediated histamine release. Regulatory T cells directly inhibit the FcγRI-dependent mast cell degranulation through cell-cell contact involving OX40-OX40L interactions between regulatory T cells and mast cells [32]. During this interaction, the concentration of cyclic adenosine monophosphate in activated mast cells is increased, leading to a reduction of calcium influx and mast cell activation. In addition, allergen-SIT decreases the influx of activated eosinophils in the tissue. It was demonstrated that allergen-SIT reduces plasma levels of eosinophil cationic protein and other chemotactic factors for eosinophils and neutrophils, which correlated with decreased bronchial hyperreactivity and clinical improvement [33]. In addition, decreased number and activation of circulating basophils have also been observed after allergen-SIT [34].

Taken together, the role of regulatory T cells in allergen-SIT is well investigated, whereas the function of other IL-10 secreting cells like monocytes or B cells and novel suppressive cytokines during SIT is still unknown.

Clinical Use

Allergen-SIT has been used for nearly 100 years as a desensitizing therapy for allergic diseases and represents a potentially curative and specific method of treatment [1]. Allergens could be administered orally during sublingual immunotherapy (SLIT), intracutaneously during subcutaneous immunotherapy, and in the lymph nodes during intralymphatic immunotherapy. Several large-scale, randomized, double blind, placebo-controlled trials demonstrated that sustained and disease-modifying effects of SLIT have been confirmed [35, 36]. Moreover, it represents high activity for novel treatment modalities, and several novel immunotherapies including oral immunotherapy for food allergy (e.g. peanut allergies) are under development [37]. SLIT depends on anatomical and functional characters of oral mucosal tissue. Oral and gastrointestinal mucosa have a natural tolerogenic character without any acute inflammation in spite of high bacterial colonization and rapid wound healing without any scar formation. Lack of inflammatory cells around mucosal tissue and high permeability for allergens suggest a way of action for sublingual allergen immunotherapy [38]. It is generally thought that the initial step of SLIT is the uptake of an allergen by Langerhans cells within the oral mucosa via high-affinity surface IgE receptors. This leads to production of IL-10 and induction of T cells with a regulatory phenotype in vitro. The mechanism of action of SLIT has been found in the same direction as in injection immunotherapy associated with increases in sublingual FOXP3-expressing cells and increased allergen-specific IgG4, IgA and serum inhibitory activity for IgE-facilitated allergen binding to B cells [39].

Although clinical trials of allergen-SIT have demonstrated treatment efficacy in various allergic diseases such as allergic asthma, allergic rhinitis, stinging insect hypersensitivity and aeroallergen-induced atopic dermatitis, there is a risk of serious adverse reactions, which can be classified in two categories: local reactions appearing as erythema, pruritus and swelling at the injection site of subcutaneous immunotherapy; and systemic reactions appearing as anaphylaxis from mild to serious life-threatening severity [40]. Moreover, repeated injections over 3 years are necessary. To improve the application of immunotherapy and reduce the risk of side effects, intralymphatic allergen administration was developed. This has enhanced safety and efficacy of immunotherapy and reduced treatment time to 8 weeks [41]. During intralymphatic immunotherapy, the vaccine is delivered directly to the lymphatic organ, which facilitates the allergen presentation by DCs to T cells compared to subcutaneous immunotherapy. In this context, new allergens that can be taken up faster and more efficiently by DCs are under development as novel treatment modalities for immunotherapy.

Conclusions

Induction of peripheral T cell tolerance by regulatory T cells is a key mechanism to suppress the excess allergic inflammation. It is characterized by induction of thymus-derived and inducible regulatory T cells, the suppressive cytokines IL-10 and TGF-β, and the noninflammatory antibody subtype IgG4. In addition, novel suppressive cell types (e.g. regulatory B cells) and cytokines (e.g. IL-35) play important roles in regulating and limiting immune reactions. Knowledge of these molecular bases is crucial to understand the regulation of the immune response and their possible therapeutic applications not only for allergic diseases, but also for other immune-related disorders such as autoimmunity, organ transplantation, malignant neoplasm and infections. In addition, novel vaccines are expected to shorten the duration, decrease the side effects and increase the efficiency of immunotherapy.

Acknowledgements

Supported by Swiss National Science Foundation grants No. 320030-132899 and 32-12549, the European Asthma and Allergy Center Davos, and CK-CARE.

References

1 Akdis CA, Akdis M: Mechanisms of allergen-specific immunotherapy. J Allergy Clin Immunol 2011;127:18–27, quiz 28–19.

2 Akdis M, Akdis CA: Therapeutic manipulation of immune tolerance in allergic disease. Nat Rev Drug Discov 2009;8:645–660.

3 Wang M, Takeda K, Shiraishi Y, Okamoto M, Dakhama A, Joetham A, Gelfand EW: Peanut-induced intestinal allergy is mediated through a mast cell-IgE-FC-epsilon-RI-IL-13 pathway. J Allergy Clin Immunol 2010;126:306–316, 316.e301–312.

4 Simons FE: Anaphylaxis. J Allergy Clin Immunol 2010;125:S161–S181.

5 Akdis M, Burgler S, Crameri R, Eiwegger T, Fujita H, Gomez E, Klunker S, Meyer N, O'Mahony L, Palomares O, Rhyner C, Quaked N, Schaffartzik A, Van De Veen W, Zeller S, Zimmermann M, Akdis CA: Interleukins, from 1 to 37, and interferon-gamma: receptors, functions, and roles in diseases. J Allergy Clin Immunol 2011;127:701–721.e1–70.

6 Solarewicz-Madejek K, Basinski TM, Crameri R, Akdis M, Akkaya A, Blaser K, Rabe KF, Akdis CA, Jutel M: T cells and eosinophils in bronchial smooth muscle cell death in asthma. Clin Exp Allergy 2009; 39:845–855.

7 Zimmermann M, Koreck A, Meyer N, Basinski T, Meiler F, Simone B, Woehrl S, Moritz K, Eiwegger T, Schmid-Grendelmeier P, Kemeny L, Akdis CA: TNF-like weak inducer of apoptosis (TWEAK) and TNF-alpha cooperate in the induction of keratinocyte apoptosis. J Allergy Clin Immunol 2011;127: 200–207, 207.e1–10.

8 Meyer N, Zimmermann M, Burgler S, Bassin C, Woehrl S, Moritz K, Rhyner C, Indermitte P, Schmid-Grendelmeier P, Akdis M, Menz G, Akdis CA: IL-32 is expressed by human primary keratinocytes and modulates keratinocyte apoptosis in atopic dermatitis. J Allergy Clin Immunol 2010;125: 858–865.e10.

9 Akkoc T, de Koning PJ, Ruckert B, Barlan I, Akdis M, Akdis CA: Increased activation-induced cell death of high IFN-gamma-producing T(h)1 cells as a mechanism of T(h)2 predominance in atopic diseases. J Allergy Clin Immunol 2008;121:652–658.e1.

10 Palomares O, Yaman G, Azkur AK, Akkoc T, Akdis M, Akdis CA: Role of Treg in immune regulation of allergic diseases. Eur J Immunol 2010;40:1232–1240.

11 Akdis M, Akdis CA: Mechanisms of allergen-specific immunotherapy. J Allergy Clin Immunol 2007;119:780–791.

12 Fontenot JD, Gavin MA, Rudensky AY: FOXP3 programs the development and function of CD4+CD25+ regulatory T cells. Nat Immunol 2003; 4:330–336.

13 Ono M, Yaguchi H, Ohkura N, Kitabayashi I, Nagamura Y, Nomura T, Miyachi Y, Tsukada T, Sakaguchi S: FOXP3 controls regulatory T-cell function by interacting with Aml1/Runx1. Nature 2007; 446:685–689.

14 Klunker S, Chong MM, Mantel PY, Palomares O, Bassin C, Ziegler M, Ruckert B, Meiler F, Akdis M, Littman DR, Akdis CA: Transcription factors Runx1 and Runx3 in the induction and suppressive function of FOXP3+ inducible regulatory T cells. J Exp Med 2009;206:2701–2715.

15 Collison LW, Workman CJ, Kuo TT, Boyd K, Wang Y, Vignali KM, Cross R, Sehy D, Blumberg RS, Vignali DA: The inhibitory cytokine IL-35 contributes to regulatory T-cell function. Nature 2007;450: 566–569.

16 Niedbala W, Wei XQ, Cai B, Hueber AJ, Leung BP, McInnes IB, Liew FY: IL-35 is a novel cytokine with therapeutic effects against collagen-induced arthritis through the expansion of regulatory T cells and suppression of Th17 cells. Eur J Immunol 2007;37: 3021–3029.

17 Collison LW, Chaturvedi V, Henderson AL, Giacomin PR, Guy C, Bankoti J, Finkelstein D, Forbes K, Workman CJ, Brown SA, Rehg JE, Jones ML, Ni HT, Artis D, Turk MJ, Vignali DA: IL-35-mediated induction of a potent regulatory T cell population. Nat Immunol 2010;11:1093–1101.

18 Ke Y, Kapp JA: Oral antigen inhibits priming of CD8+ CTL, CD4+ T cells, and antibody responses while activating CD8+ suppressor T cells. J Immunol 1996;156:916–921.

19 Chen W, Zhou D, Torrealba JR, Waddell TK, Grant D, Zhang L: Donor lymphocyte infusion induces long-term donor-specific cardiac xenograft survival through activation of recipient double-negative regulatory T cells. J Immunol 2005;175:3409–3416.

20 Deniz G, Erten G, Kucuksezer UC, Kocacik D, Karagiannidis C, Aktas E, Akdis CA, Akdis M: Regulatory NK cells suppress antigen-specific T cell responses. J Immunol 2008;180:850–857.

21 Fujita H, Teng A, Nozawa R, Takamoto-Matsui Y, Katagiri-Matsumura H, Ikezawa Z, Ishii Y: Production of both IL-27 and IFN-gamma after the treatment with a ligand for invariant NKT cells is responsible for the suppression of Th2 response and allergic inflammation in a mouse experimental asthma model. J Immunol 2009;183:254–260.

22 Ishii Y, Nozawa R, Takamoto-Matsui Y, Teng A, Katagiri-Matsumura H, Nishikawa H, Fujita H, Tamura Y: Alpha-galactosylceramide-driven immunotherapy for allergy. Front Biosci 2008;13:6214–6228.

23 Lund FE, Randall TD: Effector and regulatory B cells: modulators of CD4(+) T cell immunity. Nat Rev Immunol 2010;10:236–247.
24 Fillatreau S, Gray D, Anderton SM: Not always the bad guys: B cells as regulators of autoimmune pathology. Nat Rev Immunol 2008;8:391–397.
25 Yanaba K, Bouaziz JD, Haas KM, Poe JC, Fujimoto M, Tedder TF: A regulatory B cell subset with a unique CD1d^{hi}CD5+ phenotype controls T cell-dependent inflammatory responses. Immunity 2008; 28:639–650.
26 Iwata Y, Matsushita T, Horikawa M, Dilillo DJ, Yanaba K, Venturi GM, Szabolcs PM, Bernstein SH, Magro CM, Williams AD, Hall RP, St Clair EW, Tedder TF: Characterization of a rare IL-10-competent B-cell subset in humans that parallels mouse regulatory B10 cells. Blood 2011;117:530–541.
27 Akdis M, Verhagen J, Taylor A, Karamloo F, Karagiannidis C, Crameri R, Thunberg S, Deniz G, Valenta R, Fiebig H, Kegel C, Disch R, Schmidt-Weber CB, Blaser K, Akdis CA: Immune responses in healthy and allergic individuals are characterized by a fine balance between allergen-specific T regulatory 1 and T helper 2 cells. J Exp Med 2004;199:1567–1575.
28 Meiler F, Zumkehr J, Klunker S, Ruckert B, Akdis CA, Akdis M: In vivo switch to IL-10-secreting T regulatory cells in high dose allergen exposure. J Exp Med 2008;205:2887–2898.
29 Jutel M, Akdis M, Akdis CA: Histamine, histamine receptors and their role in immune pathology. Clin Exp Allergy 2009;39:1786–1800.
30 Platts-Mills T, Vaughan J, Squillace S, Woodfolk J, Sporik R: Sensitisation, asthma, and a modified Th2 response in children exposed to cat allergen: a population-based cross-sectional study. Lancet 2001; 357:752–756.
31 Meiler F, Klunker S, Zimmermann M, Akdis CA, Akdis M: Distinct regulation of IgE, IgG4 and IgA by T regulatory cells and Toll-like receptors. Allergy 2008;63:1455–1463.
32 Gri G, Piconese S, Frossi B, Manfroi V, Merluzzi S, Tripodo C, Viola A, Odom S, Rivera J, Colombo MP, Pucillo CE: CD4+CD25+ regulatory T cells suppress mast cell degranulation and allergic responses through OX40-OX40L interaction. Immunity 2008; 29:771–781.
33 Rak S, Hakanson L, Venge P: Immunotherapy abrogates the generation of eosinophil and neutrophil chemotactic activity during pollen season. J Allergy Clin Immunol 1990;86:706–713.
34 Shim JY, Kim BS, Cho SH, Min KU, Hong SJ: Allergen-specific conventional immunotherapy decreases immunoglobulin E-mediated basophil histamine releasability. Clin Exp Allergy 2003;33:52–57.
35 Durham SR, Emminger W, Kapp A, Colombo G, de Monchy JG, Rak S, Scadding GK, Andersen JS, Riis B, Dahl R: Long-term clinical efficacy in grass pollen-induced rhinoconjunctivitis after treatment with SQ-standardized grass allergy immunotherapy tablet. J Allergy Clin Immunol 2010;125:131–138.1–7.
36 Amar SM, Harbeck RJ, Sills M, Silveira LJ, O'Brien H, Nelson HS: Response to sublingual immunotherapy with grass pollen extract: monotherapy versus combination in a multiallergen extract. J Allergy Clin Immunol 2009;124:150–156.e1–5.
37 Crameri R, Kundig TM, Akdis CA: Modular antigen-translocation as a novel vaccine strategy for allergen-specific immunotherapy. Curr Opin Allergy Clin Immunol 2009;9:568–573.
38 Marcucci F, Incorvaia C, Sensi L, Di Cara G, Cadario G, Cavaliere A, Moingeon P, Puccinelli P, Di Gioacchino M, Frati F: Lack of inflammatory cells in the oral mucosa of subjects undergoing sublingual immunotherapy. Int J Immunopathol Pharmacol 2008;21:609–613.
39 Scadding GW, Shamji MH, Jacobson MR, Lee DI, Wilson D, Lima MT, Pitkin L, Pilette C, Nouri-Aria K, Durham SR: Sublingual grass pollen immunotherapy is associated with increases in sublingual FOXP3-expressing cells and elevated allergen-specific immunoglobulin G4, immunoglobulin A and serum inhibitory activity for immunoglobulin E-facilitated allergen binding to B cells. Clin Exp Allergy 2010;40:598–606.
40 Cox L, Larenas-Linnemann D, Lockey RF, Passalacqua G: Speaking the same language: The World Allergy Organization Subcutaneous Immunotherapy Systemic Reaction Grading System. J Allergy Clin Immunol 2010;125:569–574, 574.e1–574.e7.
41 Senti G, Prinz Vavricka BM, Erdmann I, Diaz MI, Markus R, McCormack SJ, Simard JJ, Wuthrich B, Crameri R, Graf N, Johansen P, Kundig TM: Intralymphatic allergen administration renders specific immunotherapy faster and safer: a randomized controlled trial. Proc Natl Acad Sci USA 2008;105: 17908–17912.

Dr. Cezmi A. Akdis
Swiss Institute of Allergy and Asthma Research (SIAF)
Obere Strasse 22
CH–7270 Davos (Switzerland)
Tel. +41 81 410 0848, E-Mail akdisac@siaf.uzh.ch

Ring J, Darsow U, Behrendt H (eds): New Trends in Allergy and Atopic Eczema.
Chem Immunol Allergy. Basel, Karger, 2012, vol 96, pp 39–44

Th17 and Th22 in Skin Allergy

Andrea Cavani[a] · Davide Pennino[b] · Kilian Eyerich[b]

[a]Laboratory of Experimental Immunology, IDI-IRCCS, Rome, Italy; [b]ZAUM – Center for Allergy and Environment, Technische Universität and Helmholtz Center Munich, Munich, Germany

Abstract

Development of eczematous skin reactions depends on disease-specific and time-dependent recruitment of a variety of leukocytes affecting resident skin cells through cytotoxic mechanisms and release of cytokines. Th17 and Th22, defined as RORC+IL-17+ and IL-17-IFN-γ-IL-22+ cells, respectively, belong to a newly identified class of lymphocytes specifically involved in dialogue with non-immune cells. In line with this function, both Th17 and Th22 cells are enriched in many immune-mediated skin diseases, such as atopic dermatitis, allergic contact dermatitis and psoriasis. Both IL-17 and IL-22 activate keratinocyte innate immune defenses, thus protecting the skin from pathogen invasion. However, Th17 and Th22 differ in their proinflammatory functions, being prominent in the first T cell subset and occasional/opportunistic in the second T cell subset. Most of the proinflammatory functions of Th17 depend on the synergic activity of IFN-γ and IL-17 on target cells. Together with IFN-γ, IL-17 strongly enhances adhesion molecules on keratinocytes, thus promoting T cell-keratinocyte adhesion and T cell-mediated cytotoxicity, resulting in keratinocyte apoptosis. In contrast, Th22 cells guarantee skin integrity by inducing keratinocyte proliferation and migration. However, in inflamed skin, Th22 could contribute to the amplification of immune responses by enhancing the TNF-α-induced cytokines and chemokines released by keratinocytes.

Atopic dermatitis (AD) is a chronic inflammatory skin disease that severely affects the quality of life of affected individuals [1]. The disease has a multifactorial pathogenesis, being influenced by individual genetic susceptibility, environmental factors and immunologic responses to common antigens [2–4].

The inflammatory skin infiltrate of AD lesions has been widely investigated over the last 20 years, and evidence has been provided that while Th2 cytokines prevail in the early phase of the disease, late AD is abundantly infiltrated by Th1 and Th0 cells [5–7]. Th1 cell infiltrate could have a role in the persistence of the eczematous reaction. Although CD4+ T cells greatly prevail in number, CD8+ lymphocytes can also be recruited in the early phases of the skin reaction and may contribute to induce keratinocyte apoptosis and tissue damage [8]. Recently, a role of IL-17 and IL-22 in allergic reactions has been suggested by much experimental evidence [5, 9–12]. Both cytokines are expressed in acute AD skin, and they have a major impact on epithelial cell immune functions. IL-17A is the master cytokine of Th17 lymphocytes. However, among AD infiltrating T cells, the capacity to release IL-17 is not limited to Th17, being variably expressed by a variety of tissue-derived T lymphocytes which display the capacity to produce both type 1 (IFN-γ) or type 2 (IL-4) cytokines together with IL-17. IL-22 has been originally described as a T cell-derived cytokine predominantly released by Th17 lymphocytes [13]. Indeed, most of the IL-22 released in inflamed tissue originates from a newly identified T cell subset named Th22 and from NK22, a subclass of natural killer lymphocytes that are predominantly at home in the gut [14]. Additionally, gut CD11C+ dendritic cells also produce IL-22 [15]. Although the proinflammatory role of Th17 in atopic disease has been established by a large body of experimental and clinical evidence, the contribution of Th22 lymphocytes in the disease has not been sufficiently investigated.

Th17 in Atopic Dermatitis

Th17 is a unique subset of CD4+ T lymphocytes characterized by the expression of the transcription factor RORC, the human analogue to mouse RORγt, and by the release of IL-17A and F [16–18]. Th17 may also produce variable amounts of IL-22 and IL-21. In humans, induction of Th17 phenotype is promoted by the combination of IL-1 and IL-6, which are both abundantly released during skin inflammation, whereas maintenance of the Th17 phenotype is sustained by IL-23 provided by activated dendritic cells. There is experimental evidence showing Th17 has crucial functions in host defense against pathogens and that they are involved in the pathogenesis of autoimmune skin disorders, such as psoriasis [19–21]. There is also strong evidence supporting the role of IL-17 in atopic disease, despite previous reports indicating AD is relatively poorly infiltrated by Th17 cells, as compared to psoriatic skin [22, 23]. In mice, Th17 can trigger airway inflammation, mostly mediated by neutrophil recruitment in the lung. Both AD patients and individuals with allergic asthma displayed elevated plasmatic levels of IL-17 that parallel the severity of the disease. IL-17+ cells can be detected in AD skin and at the site of the atopy patch test applied on atopic patients [9]. In the latter, the number progressively increases and reaches the maximum at 48–72 h, paralleling the expression of the eczematous reaction. Interestingly, IL-17+ T cells are mostly distributed at the site of pronounced skin damage and intense vesiculation. The majority of IL-17+ lymphocytes isolated from eczematous skin are CD4+ T lymphocytes, but they are highly heterogeneous in terms of cytokine release. Among IL-17-releasing T cells, only a fraction are pure Th17, whereas a considerable number of AD-infiltrating cells co-release IL-17 together with IL-4 or IFN-γ. Whether IL-17+IL-4+ T cells originate from Th17 or Th2 cells remains to be determined. Interestingly, both IFN-γ+IL-17+ and IL-4+IL-17+ T cells display a dual step of activation. Encounters with nominal antigens lead to full expression of IL-4 and/or IFN-γ, whereas production of IL-17 is minimal or absent. In contrast, the presence of bacterial products, such as staphylococcus-derived SEB, strongly promotes IL-17 release without further increasing IL-4 or IFN-γ. Thus SEB-producing *Staphyloccus aureus,* which colonizes AD skin, could contribute to the amplification of the inflammatory reaction by stimulating IL-17 secretion by infiltrating T cells bearing particular T cell receptor Vβ chains. A major effect of IL-17 on human keratinocytes is the induction of HBD2. However, despite availability of SEB-triggered IL-17, expression of HBD2 in AD was reported to be diminished in comparison to Th1-mediated skin immune diseases, such as psoriasis [24]. This apparent discrepancy is due to the abundant IL-4 and IL-13 in AD skin, both of which both impair the release of HBD2 by keratinocytes in response to IL-17 [9]. This could, at least in part, explain the persistent colonization of AD skin with *S. aureus*.

Besides induction of defensins, IL-17 modulates other keratinocyte innate immune responses. In particular, IL-17 promotes the release of CXCL8 and IL-6, and acts synergistically with IFN-γ to induce the expression of ICAM-1 in human keratinocytes [25, 26]. ICAM-1 is a major adhesion molecule involved in keratinocyte-T cell interaction during inflammatory skin conditions. The increased levels of ICAM-1 induced by IL-17 results in a much stronger T cell adhesiveness and consequently in an increased Fas-FasL-mediated T cell cytotoxicity towards keratinocytes. Thus, IL-17 may ultimately serve as a potent amplifier of the T cell effector mechanisms for full expression of eczematous skin reactions.

Th22 in Atopic Dermatitis

IL-22 belongs to the IL-10 cytokine family and affects target cells by binding to a heterodimeric receptor formed by IL-10R2 and the IL-22RA1 [27]. While IL-10R2 has a ubiquitous distribution, being expressed by both immune and nonimmune cells, IL-22RA1 and consequently the functional IL-22R are expressed by nonimmune cells only – epithelial cells in particular [28]. Elevated levels of IL-22 have been detected in many autoimmune diseases, and there is accumulating evidence showing that the cytokine is strongly involved in the pathogenesis of psoriasis [29]. On the other hand, a protective function of IL-22 in a murine model of hepatitis and inflammatory bowel disease has been clearly demonstrated [15, 30, 31].

Although originally described in mice as a Th17 cytokine, IL-22 is a secretion product of disparate types of leukocytes, including Th17, Th22, natural killer and LTi cells, as well as CD11c dendritic cells [32, 33]. Th22 is a recently identified novel T cell subset showing a pronounced attitude to infiltrate the skin under inflammatory conditions and is characterized by the release of IL-22 and TNF-α, but not IL-17, IL-4 and IFN-γ [10, 34, 35]. When compared to Th1, Th2 and Th17 cells, skin Th22 cells show a unique profile of gene expression that comprises several fibroblast growth factors and the chemokines CCL-7, CCL-15 and CCL-23.

Similarly to what has been observed for IL-17+ T cells, not all the IL-22+ T cells infiltrating AD skin belong to the Th22 subset since variable, but significant, amounts of IL-22 can be released by Th17, Th1 and, to a lesser extent, Th2 lymphocytes. Additionally, a variable number of CD3+CD8+ T cells isolated from various inflammatory skin diseases also release IL-22.

Th22 cells have multiple effects on keratinocytes. Transcriptome analysis of human keratinocytes treated in vitro with supernatants of activated Th22 cells revealed the induction of several chemokines, cytokines, defensins, Toll-like receptors 3 and 6, and complement components. CXCL9, 10 and 11, which direct the recruitment of Th1 and Tc1 cells into the skin, are strongly upregulated in keratinocytes exposed in vitro to Th22 supernatants. IL-7 and IL-15 are survival cytokines for T and natural killer lymphocytes. Defensins and Toll-like receptor expression are critical for keratinocyte innate responses against pathogens. Most of these proinflammatory effects of Th22 cells are dependent on the simultaneous release of TNF-α by Th22. In contrast, regenerative and protective functions of Th22 cells mostly depend on IL-22 alone or together with fibroblast growth factor release. IL-22 affects keratinocyte via the STAT3 signal pathway, augmenting cell proliferation and migration, as well as reducing keratinocyte differentiation. Thus, besides the proinflammatory function, which is mostly dependent on the combined secretion of IL-22 and TNF-α, the major role of Th22 in peripheral tissues is to guarantee the integrity of epithelia following injuries or inflammatory processes that may alter the barrier function of the skin.

Taken together, the data indicate a dual role of Th22 in skin inflammation. The protective/regenerative function and the proinflammatory function of Th22 are primarily involved in the maintenance of skin homeostasis, although in certain situations, activation of Th22 may be detrimental and may contribute to disease expression.

Conclusions

Th17 and Th22 cells belong to a new class of tissue-signaling T lymphocytes that are critically involved in directing innate immune responses in peripheral tissues. Despite the overlapping functions aimed at protecting peripheral tissues from pathogens, the biological significance of Th17 and Th22 appears quite distinct. Th17 cells protect the skin by promoting inflammation, by facilitating neutrophils and T cell recruitment, and finally by enhancing T cell effector functions. In contrast, Th22 cells have limited inflammatory properties, but guarantee skin homeostasis mostly by contrasting pathogen entry in the organism, thanks to their capacity to induce epithelial cell proliferation and migration.

References

1 Leung DY, Boguniewicz M, Howell MD, Nomura I, Hamid QA: New insights into atopic dermatitis. J Clin Invest 2004;113:651–657.

2 Jutel M, Akdis CA: T-cell subset regulation in atopy. Curr Allergy Asthma Rep 2011;11:139–145.

3 Albanesi C: Keratinocytes in allergic skin diseases. Curr Opin Allergy Clin Immunol 2010;10:452–456.

4 Guttman-Yassky E, Suarez-Farinas M, Chiricozzi A, Nograles KE, Shemer A, et al: Broad defects in epidermal cornification in atopic dermatitis identified through genomic analysis. J Allergy Clin Immunol 2009;124:1235–1244 e1258.

5 Akdis M: The cellular orchestra in skin allergy; are differences to lung and nose relevant? Curr Opin Allergy Clin Immunol 2010;10:443–451.

6 Guttman-Yassky E, Nograles KE, Krueger JG: Contrasting pathogenesis of atopic dermatitis and psoriasis – part I: clinical and pathologic concepts. J Allergy Clin Immunol 2011;127:1110–1118.

7 Guttman-Yassky E, Nograles KE, Krueger JG: Contrasting pathogenesis of atopic dermatitis and psoriasis – part II: immune cell subsets and therapeutic concepts. J Allergy Clin Immunol 2011;127:1420–1432.

8 Hennino A, Jean-Decoster C, Giordano-Labadie F, Debeer S, Vanbervliet B, et al: CD8+ T cells are recruited early to allergen exposure sites in atopy patch test reactions in human atopic dermatitis. J Allergy Clin Immunol 2011;127:1064–1067.

9 Eyerich K, Pennino D, Scarponi C, Foerster S, Nasorri F, et al: IL-17 in atopic eczema: linking allergen-specific adaptive and microbial-triggered innate immune response. J Allergy Clin Immunol 2009;123:59–66.e54.

10 Eyerich S, Eyerich K, Pennino D, Carbone T, Nasorri F, et al: Th22 cells represent a distinct human T cell subset involved in epidermal immunity and remodeling. J Clin Invest 2009;119:3573–3585.

11 Koga C, Kabashima K, Shiraishi N, Kobayashi M, Tokura Y: Possible pathogenic role of Th17 cells for atopic dermatitis. J Invest Dermatol 2008;128:2625–2630.

12 Souwer Y, Szegedi K, Kapsenberg ML, de Jong EC: IL-17 and IL-22 in atopic allergic disease. Curr Opin Immunol 2010;22:821–826.

13 Liang SC, Tan XY, Luxenberg DP, Karim R, Dunussi-Joannopoulos K, et al: Interleukin (IL)-22 and IL-17 are coexpressed by Th17 cells and cooperatively enhance expression of antimicrobial peptides. J Exp Med 2006;203:2271–2279.

14 Cella M, Fuchs A, Vermi W, Facchetti F, Otero K, et al: A human natural killer cell subset provides an innate source of IL-22 for mucosal immunity. Nature 2009;457:722–725.

15 Zenewicz LA, Yancopoulos GD, Valenzuela DM, Murphy AJ, Stevens S, et al: Innate and adaptive interleukin-22 protects mice from inflammatory bowel disease. Immunity 2008;29:947–957.

16 Burgler S, Ouaked N, Bassin C, Basinski TM, Mantel PY, et al: Differentiation and functional analysis of human T(H)17 cells. J Allergy Clin Immunol 2009;123:588–595, 595.e1–7.

17 Acosta-Rodriguez EV, Rivino L, Geginat J, Jarrossay D, Gattorno M, et al: Surface phenotype and antigenic specificity of human interleukin 17-producing T helper memory cells. Nat Immunol 2007;8:639–646.

18 Korn T, Bettelli E, Oukka M, Kuchroo VK: IL-17 and Th17 cells. Ann Rev Immunol 2009;27:485–517.

19 Bettelli E, Oukka M, Kuchroo VK: T(H)-17 cells in the circle of immunity and autoimmunity. Nat Immunol 2007;8:345–350.

20 Zaba LC, Fuentes-Duculan J, Eungdamrong NJ, Abello MV, Novitskaya I, et al: Psoriasis is characterized by accumulation of immunostimulatory and Th1/Th17 cell-polarizing myeloid dendritic cells. J Invest Dermatol 2009;129:79–88.

21 Eyerich K, Foerster S, Rombold S, Seidl HP, Behrendt H, et al: Patients with chronic mucocutaneous candidiasis exhibit reduced production of Th17-associated cytokines IL-17 and IL-22. J Invest Dermatol 2008;128:2640–2645.

22 Guttman-Yassky E, Lowes MA, Fuentes-Duculan J, Zaba LC, Cardinale I, et al: Low expression of the IL-23/Th17 pathway in atopic dermatitis compared to psoriasis. J Immunol 2008;181:7420–7427.

23 Irving K: Asthma and allergy: complementing the IL-17 axis in asthma. Nat Rev Immunol 2010;10:676.

24 Ong PY, Ohtake T, Brandt C, Strickland I, Boguniewicz M, et al: Endogenous antimicrobial peptides and skin infections in atopic dermatitis. N Engl J Med 2002;347:1151–1160.

25 Albanesi C, Cavani A, Girolomoni G: IL-17 is produced by nickel-specific T lymphocytes and regulates ICAM-1 expression and chemokine production in human keratinocytes: synergistic or antagonist effects with IFN-gamma and TNF-alpha. J Immunol 1999;162:494–502.

26 Pennino D, Eyerich K, Scarponi C, Carbone T, Eyerich S, et al: IL-17 amplifies human contact hypersensitivity by licensing hapten nonspecific Th1 cells to kill autologous keratinocytes. J Immunol 2010;184:4880–4888.

27 Kotenko SV, Izotova LS, Mirochnitchenko OV, Esterova E, Dickensheets H, et al: Identification of the functional interleukin-22 (IL-22) receptor complex: the IL-10R2 chain (IL-10Rbeta) is a common chain of both the IL-10 and IL-22 (IL-10-related T cell-derived inducible factor, IL-TIF) receptor complexes. J Biol Chem 2001;276:2725–2732.
28 Wolk K, Kunz S, Witte E, Friedrich M, Asadullah K, et al: IL-22 increases the innate immunity of tissues. Immunity 2004;21:241–254.
29 Zheng Y, Danilenko DM, Valdez P, Kasman I, Eastham-Anderson J, et al: Interleukin-22, a T(H)17 cytokine, mediates IL-23-induced dermal inflammation and acanthosis. Nature 2007;445:648–651.
30 Zheng Y, Valdez PA, Danilenko DM, Hu Y, Sa SM, et al: Interleukin-22 mediates early host defense against attaching and effacing bacterial pathogens. Nat Med 2008;14:282–289.
31 Zenewicz LA, Yancopoulos GD, Valenzuela DM, Murphy AJ, Karow M, et al: Interleukin-22 but not interleukin-17 provides protection to hepatocytes during acute liver inflammation. Immunity 2007;27:647–659.
32 Vivier E, Spits H, Cupedo T: Interleukin-22-producing innate immune cells: new players in mucosal immunity and tissue repair? Nat Rev Immunol 2009;9:229–234.
33 Eyerich S, Eyerich K, Cavani A, Schmidt-Weber C: IL-17 and IL-22: siblings, not twins. Trends Immunol 2010;31:354–361.
34 Trifari S, Kaplan CD, Tran EH, Crellin NK, Spits H: Identification of a human helper T cell population that has abundant production of interleukin 22 and is distinct from T(H)-17, T(H)1 and T(H)2 cells. Nat Immunol 2009;10:864–871.
35 Duhen T, Geiger R, Jarrossay D, Lanzavecchia A, Sallusto F: Production of interleukin 22 but not interleukin 17 by a subset of human skin-homing memory T cells. Nature Immunol 2009;10:857–863.

Dr. Andrea Cavani
Laboratory of Experimental Immunology, IDI-IRCCS
Via Dei Monti di Creta 104
IT–00167 Rome (Italy)
Tel. +39 06 6646 4775, E-Mail Cavini@idi.it

Ring J, Darsow U, Behrendt H (eds): New Trends in Allergy and Atopic Eczema.
Chem Immunol Allergy. Basel, Karger, 2012, vol 96, pp 45–49

IL-25 Induces Both Inflammation and Skin Barrier Dysfunction in Atopic Dermatitis

Mette Deleuran[a] · Malene Hvid[b] · Kaare Kemp[c] ·
Gitte B. Christensen[c] · Bent Deleuran[b] · Christian Vestergaard[a]

[a]Department of Dermatology, Aarhus University Hospital, [b]Department of Medical Microbiology and Immunology, Aarhus University, Aarhus, [c]LEO Pharma, Ballerup, Denmark

Abstract

Atopic dermatitis (AD) is a chronic relapsing skin disease characterized by having both an epidermal and a dermal component, shown as a barrier deficiency and inflammation. The mechanisms resulting in skewing the immune response in a Th2 direction in AD are still not fully elucidated. We suggest that IL-25 could be a major target in AD. IL-25 is produced by cells within the dermis of AD patients, and we suggest these to be dendritic cells (DCs). Furthermore, we show that IL-25 can inhibit filaggrin synthesis in keratinocytes. These results point towards a central role of IL-25 producing DCs that can induce both a Th2 response and inhibit filaggrin synthesis. We believe this strongly supports a role for IL-25 in AD, bridging the gap between inflammation and impaired skin barrier function.

In searching for new ways to understand the pathogenesis of atopic dermatitis (AD), one must consider the simple facts that AD has both an epidermal and a dermal component, shown as a barrier deficiency and inflammation.

Th2 cells and Th2-associated cytokines are considered pivotal for the development of AD, and increased levels of the Th2-associated cytokines IL-4, IL-5 and IL-13 are present, especially in the acute phase of the disease. Further, it has recently been demonstrated that a significant proportion of patients with AD carry null mutations in the keratinocyte-derived protein filaggrin which are associated with impaired skin barrier function [1].

IL-25 is a newly identified cytokine belonging to the IL-17 family. Due to this relationship, IL-25 is also known as IL-17E. The biological effects of IL-25 are mediated through IL-17RB (also known as IL-17Rh1 or IL-17 BR) and IL-17RA, two members of the IL-17 receptor family. Although IL-25 does not bind to IL-17RA, this receptor seems to be necessary for activating signals in response to IL-25 [2, 3].

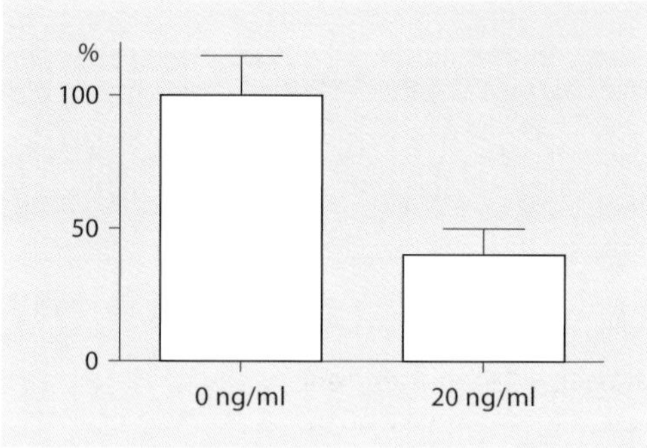

Fig. 1. IL-25 suppresses filaggrin synthesis in cultured keratinocytes. Primary keratinocytes were cultured with and without IL-25, showing a significant reduction in filaggrin mRNA synthesis by QRT-PCR.

IL-25 participates in the initiation and prolongation of Th2-directed immune responses in murine models [4], and protein and mRNA levels of this cytokine have been shown to be elevated in the lungs of asthmatic patients. Furthermore, IL-25 administration induces the production of the Th2-associated cytokines IL-4, IL-5 and IL-13 in addition to eosinophilia and IgE production in a murine model of asthma [5]. Th2 cells, mast cells and lung epithelial cells are among the cell types producing the cytokine [5–7].

Additionally, it has been shown earlier that expression levels of both IL-25 and its receptor are elevated in human AD lesions [8].

We therefore examined if IL-25 could play a central role in AD, both concerning the inflammatory component and the barrier dysfunction [9].

We started out by studying AD skin biopsies for the amount of IL-25 mRNA synthesis, and found that it was very low and just above the detection limit, but still higher in AD skin than in samples from healthy volunteers. This was in contrast to results obtained by immunohistochemistry, where we observed IL-25 in keratinocytes in involved, but also less intensely in uninvolved skin from AD patients, and with IL-17RB coexpressed primarily along the basal membrane in the involved skin. This turned our attention to the dermis where large mononuclear cells abundantly expressed IL-25, with a few also expressing IL-17RB. Uninvolved skin and healthy control skin showed signs of the same pattern, but much less pronounced.

Combining the knowledge from these different experiments led us to speculate whether IL-25 is produced primarily by a cell type that is not stationary, but migrates into the skin.

Due to the morphology of the IL-25-producing cells in the dermis, we suggested that dendritic cells (DCs) could be responsible for most of the IL-25 production observed. In order to pursue this hypothesis, we transformed peripheral blood monocytes into dendritic cells (mDC) [9]. We then investigated these cells for the presence of IL-25 and its receptor IL-17RB, demonstrating that approximately one third of the unstimulated mDCs produced IL-25, whereas IL-17RB was present on approximately

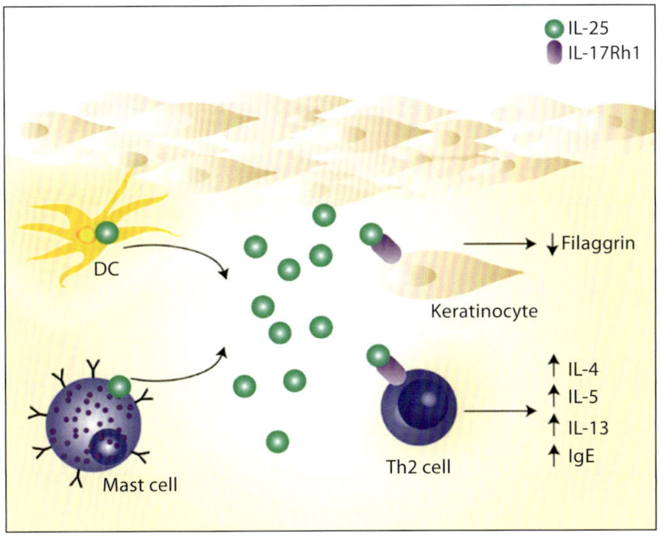

Fig. 2. The role of IL-25 in atopic dermatitis. IL-25 is produced by dermal dendritic cells and can induce a Th2 response, stimulate mast cell degranulation and inhibit filaggrin synthesis. All these features are central issues in the pathogenesis of atopic dermatitis, supporting that IL-25 is pivotal for this disease.

3% of the cells. Since secondary infections are common in AD, we further investigated the effect of lipopolysaccharide (LPS) stimulation on IL-25 production by the mDCs. LPS induced a significant increase in the number of IL-25-producing mDCs, whereas the number of IL-17RB-expressing cells was unchanged. Stimulation with thymus stromal lymphopoietin (TSLP) did not show any effect.

Keratinocytes are the predominant cell type present in the epidermis, and they produce the protein filaggrin. Under normal conditions, this protein is degraded into smaller molecules known as natural moisturizing factors (NMF), which are important for the intact barrier function found in normal skin. Null mutations in the gene coding for filaggrin is associated with a lack of NMF, leading to dry skin and barrier dysfunction, and it has recently been observed that a significant proportion of patients suffering from AD carry such mutations. This does however not explain why all patients with AD have a skin barrier dysfunction. We therefore examined whether IL-25 could affect filaggrin synthesis in primary keratinocyte cultures. We found that IL-25 stimulation significantly reduced the mRNA synthesis of filaggrin in a dose-dependent manner, supporting that IL-25 also has a direct effect on skin barrier function.

Conclusion and Perspectives

In our understanding of AD, the report of mutations in the gene encoding filaggrin as a genetic disposition for development of the disease was a huge step forward. However, it is only present in approximately 20% of patients suffering from the condition. Secondly, we have known for years that both an epidermal and dermal component is present, shown as a barrier deficiency and inflammation. Furthermore, the filaggrin defect does not explain why we observe a Th2 response in the acute phase of the disease.

IL-25 is connected to the development of a Th2 response [4], and we report the presence of IL-25 in AD skin, suggesting that DCs could be important in this perspective. We believe the link to AD is strengthened by the fact that LPS increases IL-25 production and receptor expression. We could only detect very low levels of IL-25 mRNA in skin biopsies from AD patients. Therefore, although IL-25 expression was present in the epidermal keratinocytes, it seemed as if it was synthesized elsewhere. This could be explained by the migration of IL-25-producing DCs into the inflamed tissue. Furthermore, keratinocytes have previously been shown to have a very low level of synthesis of other cytokines [10].

We suggest that DC could play an important role in the skewing of the immune response towards Th2 in AD and at the same time alter the synthesis of filaggrin, especially as DCs are present in AD skin in increased numbers.

T cells, and to some extent mast cells/basophils have up to now been considered to be the main inducers of a Th2 profile, but the discovery of IL-25 in the epidermis suggests that keratinocytes can themselves facilitate a Th2 response. That DC also have this ability suggests that the antigen-presenting cell can inflict this response, opening up a whole new possibility to interact with the immune mechanisms.

We propose a role for IL-25 in AD in bridging the gap between inflammation and impaired skin barrier function of the epidermis, and our results suggest that keratinocytes and DCs may also play a pivotal role in AD. This helps to explain why we see both epidermal and dermal changes in AD, as IL-25 possesses the ability to induce both impaired barrier function and Th2-like inflammation.

References

1 Palmer CN, Irvine AD, Terron-Kwiatkowski A, Zhao Y, Liao H, Lee SP, Goudie DR, Sandilands A, Campbell LE, Smith FJ, O'Regan GM, Watson RM, Cecil JE, Bale SJ, Compton JG, DiGiovanna JJ, Fleckman P, Lewis-Jones S, Arseculeratne G, Sergeant A, Munro CS, El Houate B, McElreavey K, Halkjaer LB, Bisgaard H, Mukhopadhyay S, McLean WH: Common loss-of-function variants of the epidermal barrier protein filaggrin are a major predisposing factor for atopic dermatitis. Nat Genet 2006; 38:441–446.

2 Rickel EA, Siegel LA, Yoon BR, Rottman JB, Kugler DG, Swart DA, Anders PM, Tocker JE, Comeau MR, Budelsky AL: Identification of functional roles for both IL-17RB and IL-17RA in mediating IL-25-induced activities. J Immunol 2008;181:4299–4310.

3 Lee J, Ho WH, Maruoka M, Corpuz RT, Baldwin DT, Foster JS, Goddard AD, Yansura DG, Vandlen RL, Wood WI, Gurney AL: IL-17E, a novel proinflammatory ligand for the IL-17 receptor homolog IL-17Rh1. J Biol Chem 2001;276:1660–1664.

4 Hurst SD, Muchamuel T, Gorman DM, Gilbert JM, Clifford T, Kwan S, Menon S, Seymour B, Jackson C, Kung TT, Brieland JK, Zurawski SM, Chapman RW, Zurawski G, Coffman RL: New IL-17 family members promote Th1 or Th2 responses in the lung: in vivo function of the novel cytokine IL-25. J Immunol 2002;169:443–453.

5 Fort MM, Cheung J, Yen D, Li J, Zurawski SM, Lo S, Menon S, Clifford T, Hunte B, Lesley R, Muchamuel T, Hurst SD, Zurawski G, Leach MW, Gorman DM, Rennick DM: IL-25 induces IL-4, IL-5, and IL-13 and Th2-associated pathologies in vivo. Immunity 2001;15:985–995.
6 Angkasekwinai P, Park H, Wang YH, Wang YH, Chang SH, Corry DB, Liu YJ, Zhu Z, Dong C: Interleukin 25 promotes the initiation of proallergic type 2 responses. J Exp Med 2007;204:1509–1517.
7 Ikeda K, Nakajima H, Suzuki K, Kagami S, Hirose K, Suto A, Saito Y, Iwamoto I: Mast cells produce interleukin-25 upon Fc epsilon RI-mediated activation. Blood 2003;101:3594–3596.
8 Wang YH, Angkasekwinai P, Lu N, Voo KS, Arima K, Hanabuchi S, Hippe A, Corrigan CJ, Dong C, Homey B, Yao Z, Ying S, Huston DP, Liu YJ: IL-25 augments type 2 immune responses by enhancing the expansion and functions of TSLP-DC-activated Th2 memory cells. J Exp Med 2007;204:1837–1847.
9 Hvid M, Vestergaard C, Kemp K, Christensen GB, Deleuran B, Deleuran M: IL-25 in atopic dermatitis: a possible link between inflammation and skin barrier dysfunction? J Invest Dermatol 2011;131:150–157.
10 Kristensen MS, Paludan K, Larsen CG, Zachariae CO, Deleuran BW, Jensen PK, Jørgensen P, Thestrup-Pedersen K: Quantitative determination of IL-1 alpha-induced IL-8 mRNA levels in cultured human keratinocytes, dermal fibroblasts, endothelial cells, and monocytes. J Invest Dermatol 1991;97: 506–510.

Dr. Mette Deleuran
Department of Dermatology, Aarhus University Hospital
P.P. Ørums Gade 11
DK–8000 Aarhus C (Denmark)
Tel. +45 8949 1851, E-Mail mettdele@rm.dk

Ring J, Darsow U, Behrendt H (eds): New Trends in Allergy and Atopic Eczema.
Chem Immunol Allergy. Basel, Karger, 2012, vol 96, pp 50–60

Angiogenesis, Lymphangiogenesis and Atopic Dermatitis

A. Genovese · A. Detoraki · F. Granata · M.R. Galdiero · G. Spadaro · G. Marone

Department of Clinical Immunology and Allergy and Center for Basic and Clinical Immunology Research (CISI), University of Naples Federico II, Naples, Italy

Abstract

Angiogenesis and morphological and functional alterations of microvessels are hallmark features of chronic inflammatory disorders, including certain skin diseases. Vascular endothelial growth factors (VEGFs) are key regulators of blood vessel growth. The VEGF family includes VEGF-A, -B, -C, -D and placental growth factor. VEGF-A and -B are the most important proangiogenic factors, while VEGF-C and -D primarily regulate lymphangiogenesis. Angiopoietins are promoters of neovascularization by interacting with Tie-1 and Tie-2 receptors present on endothelial cells. High levels of VEGF-A have been detected in skin tissue of atopic dermatitis (AD) patients and correlate with disease activity. The vascular changes in the skin of AD patients appear to be linked to the inflammatory process. Effector cells of skin inflammation (human mast cells, basophils, eosinophils, macrophages, lymphocytes, etc.) are major sources of a vast array of angiogenic and lymphangiogenic factors. The role of lymphangiogenesis in AD is largely unknown.

Blood vessels arise from endothelial progenitors which assemble in a vascular labyrinth of small capillaries, in a process known as vasculogenesis [1]. Nascent endothelial cell (EC) channels become covered by pericytes and smooth muscle cells, which provide strength and allow regulation of vessel perfusion; this is arteriogenesis. The lymphatic system develops in parallel but secondarily to the blood vascular system through a process known as lymphangiogenesis [2].

Angiogenesis, a term coined by John Hunter in 1787, contributes to organ growth during early life; however, during adult life, blood vessels remain quiescent and angiogenesis occurs only in the cycling ovary and in the placenta [1, 2]. Angiogenesis in the skin is reactivated during wound healing and repair [3, 4]. In these settings several angiogenic factors are released by activated keratinocytes and other cell types including several inflammatory cells [5–7]. In certain disorders, these stimuli become excessive and the balance between stimulators and inhibitors shifts, resulting in a (lymph)angiogenic switch. The best known conditions in which this switch is seen are malignant and inflammatory skin disorders [3].

Proangiogenic Factors

Vascular endothelial growth factor (VEGF), previously known as vascular permeability factor [8] is the most specific growth factor for vascular endothelium [1]. The VEGF family includes VEGF-A, -B, -C, -D, and placental growth factor (PlGF) [1, 9]. VEGF-A and -B are key regulators of blood vessel growth, while VEGF-C and -D primarily regulate lymphangiogenesis [2]. Human VEGF-A has at least six isoforms (121, 145, 165, 183, 189 and 204) that differ in their effects on angiogenesis. VEGF-A_{165} is the most potent proangiogenic isoform [10]. PlGF, expressed in the placenta and certain tumors, has two major isoforms: PlGF-1($PlGF_{131}$) and PlGF-2 ($PlGF_{152}$) [11].

VEGFs signal through three human VEGF receptors (VEGFR): VEGFR-1, VEGFR-2 and VEGFR-3 [1]. VEGF functions are also regulated through the production of an alternative mRNA variant of VEGFR-1, soluble VEGFR-1. Neuropilin-1 (NRP-1) and NRP-2 are co-receptors for VEGF [12, 13]. NRP-1 is expressed by arterial EC [14], and NRP-2 is expressed by venous and lymphatic EC [15]. NRP-1 boosts the affinity of VEGF-A_{165} for VEGFR-2 [13] and increases its phosphorylation, enhancing downstream signaling [16] (fig. 1).

Other naturally occurring promoters of embryonic and postnatal neovascularization are angiopoietins (Angs) which interact with Tie-1 and Tie-2 receptors. In humans, Ang-1 promotes angiogenesis by establishing and maintaining vascular integrity and quiescence [17]. Ang-1 binds the Tie-2 receptor [18], whereas Ang-2 reduces vascular integrity by competing for Tie-2. No ligand has been identified for Tie-1, which is currently considered an orphan receptor. Ang-1 is widely expressed in normal adult tissues, whereas Ang-2 is expressed mainly at sites of vascular remodeling such as chronic inflammation [19] (fig. 2). The role of Angs in lymphangiogenesis is not clear. However, Ang-1 overexpression induces lymphatic vessel enlargement, sprouting and proliferation [20].

Angiogenin, normally present in the circulation, is one of the most potent tumor-derived angiogenic factors and plays a role in a number of nonmalignant vasculoproliferative pathologies [21]. Angiogenin is produced by macrophages, EC and lymphocytes [22].

Basic fibroblast growth factor (FGF-β) stimulates EC proliferation and migration in vitro and angiogenesis in vivo [23]. FGF-β plays a significant role in inflammatory conditions, including wound healing and fibrosis, and its tissue distribution suggests a role in angiogenesis [24].

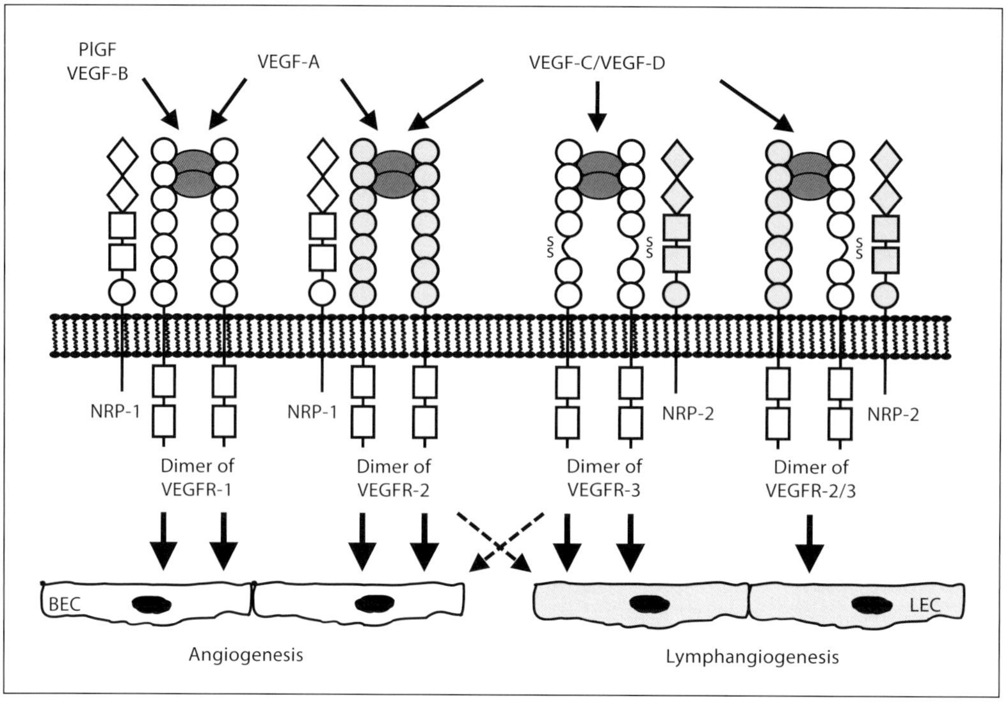

Fig. 1. Schematic representation of the family of VEGF and their receptors. This family of structurally related molecules includes VEGF-A, -B,- C, -D and PlGF. VEGF-A is the main mediator of angiogenesis. The VEGFs form antiparallel dimers that induce dimerization and activation of their cognate receptors on binding. VEGFR-1 and VEGFR-2 are composed of seven Ig-like domains (circles) and a split tyrosine kinase (rectangles). The fifth Ig-like domain of VEGFR-3 is proteolitically cleaved. VEGF-A activates tyrosine kinase receptors VEGFR-1 and VEGFR-2. VEGF-A signals mainly through VEGFR-2, which is expressed at high levels by blood vascular endothelial cells (BEC). VEGF-B and PlGF specifically activate VEGFR-1. VEGFR-2 is also found in lymphatic vascular endothelial cells (LEC) and VEGFR-2/3 heterodimers may form in these cells. VEGF-C and -D activate VEGFR-3 and VEGFR-2. VEGFR-3 is largely expressed by LEC. Besides the three tyrosine-kinase receptors, there are coreceptors for VEGFs such as neuropilins (NRPs). NRP-1 associates with VEGFR-1 and VEGFR-2 to bind VEGF-A_{165}, VEGF-B, and PlGF. NRP-2 associates with VEGFR-3 to bind VEGF-C and VEGF-D to regulate lymphangiogenesis.

Several cytokines and chemokines are involved in angiogenesis. IL-8, produced by monocytes, macrophages and mast cells, is a potent mediator of angiogenesis [25]. IL-8 has at least four distinct proangiogenic properties: it boosts EC proliferation, induces EC chemotaxis and survival, and activates proteases [26].

IL-17, produced mainly by a subset of activated $CD4^+$ T cells (Th17) [27], mediates angiogenesis in humans by stimulating EC migration and cord formation, and regulating the production of a variety of proangiogenic factors [28]. Promotion of angiogenesis by IL-17 may result from enhancement of the action of the FGF-β, the hepatocyte growth factor and VEGF [29].

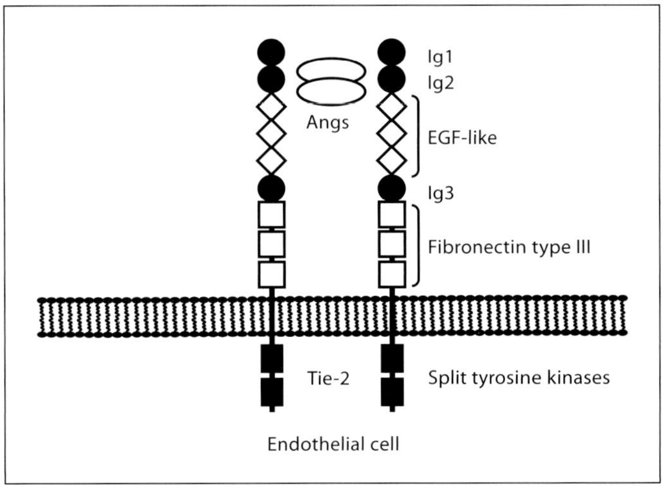

Fig. 2. Schematic representation of Angs and Tie-2 receptor. Angs are structurally related endothelial growth factors, with similar binding affinity for the tyrosine kinase receptor Tie-2. Tie-2 is composed of three Ig-like domains (Ig1, Ig2 and Ig3; circles) separated by two EGF-like domains (rhombs), three fibronectin type III domains (open squares) and a split tyrosine kinase (closed squares). Ang-1 forms dimers that induce dimerization and activation of Tie-2 receptor and binding. Ang-1 acts as a Tie-2 agonist, promoting EC survival, migration and proliferation, Ang-2 is an endogenous Tie-2 antagonist, thereby counteracting Ang-1 activities. Tie-2 is also found on human neutrophils, mouse and human mast cells, and mouse monocytes.

Angiogenic Factors in Atopic Dermatitis

AD is a common inflammatory skin disease characterized by a chronic relapsing form of skin inflammation, a disturbance of epidermal-barrier function that culminates in dry skin, and IgE-mediated sensitization to food and environmental allergens [30–32]. The histologic features of acute eczematous patches and plaques are epidermal intercellular edema (spongiosis) and a prominent perivascular infiltrate of lymphocytes, monocyte/macrophages, dendritic cells and a few eosinophils in the dermis. In subacute and chronic lichenified and excoriated plaques, the epidermis is thickened and its upper layer is hypertrophied.

The clinical manifestations of AD vary with age. In infancy, the first eczematous lesions usually emerge on the cheeks and the scalp. During childhood, lesions involve flexures, the nape and the dorsal aspects of the limbs. In adolescence and adulthood, lichenified plaques affect the flexures, head and neck. In each stage, itching that worsens at night causes sleep loss and substantially impairs the patient's quality of life [30].

Skin tissue remodeling is a central feature of several inflammatory skin disorders (psoriasis, AD, etc.). Although vascular remodeling has been extensively studied in psoriasis [33, 34], this aspect has been largely neglected in AD. The concentrations of VEGF in plasma of AD patients are slightly increased compared to healthy controls [35]. Normal keratinocytes moderately express VEGF, but cultured keratinocytes release this angiogenic factor [36]. During wound repair, VEGF is abundantly produced by skin keratinocytes [37]. Human keratinocytes express VEGFR-1 [38], VEGFR-2, VEGFR-3 and neuropilins [39]. Interestingly, VEGF enhances the proliferation and migration of keratinocytes, presumably by binding to VEGFR-2 [39]. Finally, VEGF in the stratum corneum of lesional scars of AD patients are markedly increased compared to the patients' healthy skin tissue [40].

Recently, an association between the –1154 G/A promoter polymorphism of the VEGF gene and AD was reported in Polish patients [41]. The functional effect of these polymorphisms is presently unclear and further investigations in larger groups and different populations are needed.

Cellular Sources of Angiogenic and Lymphangiogenic Factors in Atopic Dermatitis

Keratinocytes and possibly other stromal cells can be a source of angiogenic factors during wound healing and scar formation. In addition, there is increasing evidence that inflammatory cells that participate in the pathogenesis of AD [30, 33, 34] represent a significant source of angiogenic and lymphangiogenic factors [6, 7, 42–44].

Mast cells are in close proximity to EC in the epidermis of AD lesions [43]. The same group of investigators demonstrated that human skin mast cells contain and release VEGF-A [44]. We have demonstrated that primary human mast cells constitutively produce, in addition to VEGF-A, angiogenic VEGF-B and lymphangiogenic VEGF-C and -D [6]. These factors are probably preformed in mast cells since VEGF-A, VEGF-C and VEGF-D can be detected by immunostaining. Interestingly, two inflammatory stimuli, PGE_2 and adenosine, induce the expression of both angiogenic (VEGF-A and -B) and lymphangiogenic (-C and -D) VEGFs in human mast cells and elicit the release of VEGF-A in mast cell supernatants, which in turn induce an angiogenic response in the chorioallantoic membrane system [6]. Collectively, these findings indicate that human mast cells have an intrinsic capacity to produce several VEGFs, suggesting that these cells might modulate both angiogenesis and lymphangiogenesis in AD.

Mast cells appear to be not only a source of VEGFs in the skin, but also a target for these factors. In fact, human mast cells express VEGFR-1 and -2 which are the major receptors for the VEGFs. In addition, we have demonstrated that different VEGFs (VEGF-A, -B, -C, -D and PlGF-1) exert chemotactic effects on mast cells by engaging both receptors. Since there is evidence that mast cells accumulate at sites of angiogenesis [45], it is possible that VEGFs produced by mast cells and other resident cells exert paracrine recruitment of mast cells in the skin, thereby sustaining both inflammatory and angiogenic processes.

Macrophages are also relevant to the pathogenesis of AD [30]. Activated macrophages induce neovascularization and contribute to angiogenesis and lymphangiogenesis in inflammatory diseases and cancer. Primary human macrophages express angiogenic (VEGF-A and -B) and lymphangiogenic factors (VEGF-C and -D) [7]. Secretory phospholipases A_2, enzymes present in the sites of inflammation [46], enhance the expression and release of VEGF-A and -C [7].

Eosinophils may be involved in regulating angiogenesis in AD. Eosinophils synthesize and store in their granules several proangiogenic mediators such as VEGF-A, FGF-2, TNF-α, GM-CSF, NGF and IL-8. In addition, these cells promote EC proliferation in vitro and induce new vessel formation in aortic rings and in the chorioallantoic membrane [47].

Basophils, primary effector cells in allergic inflammation, produce several forms of VEGF-A (121, 165, 189) and VEGF-B (167, 186), and their secretory granules contain VEGF-A [5]. IgE-mediated activation of these cells caused VEGF-A release and supernatants of activated basophils induced an angiogenic response in vivo. $VEGF\text{-}A_{165}$ has a chemotactic effect on basophils through the activation of VEGFR-2. Since these cells do not express VEGF-C and -D, circulating basophils presumably play a role in neoangiogenesis, but not in lymphangiogenesis.

The Ang/Tie receptors system is known to interact with the VEGF/VEGFR pathway to determine the fate of blood vessels during angiogenesis [48]. Recently, it has been reported that VEGF, Ang-1, Ang-2 and Tie-2 are increased in human dermal wound repair and scarring [4]. Interestingly, we have shown that activated basophils release Ang-1 that exerts chemotactic activity on human mast cells through the interaction with Tie-2 receptor (Prevete et al., personal communication).

IL-17-producing $CD4^+$ T helper cells (Th17 cells) have a crucial role in host defense, and dysregulated Th17 cell responses mediate a variety of inflammatory and autoimmune disorders [49]. There is evidence that IL-17 promotes angiogenesis directly [50] and by enhancing the production of angiogenic chemokines [28] or VEGF [51]. $IL\text{-}17^+$ cells are present in skin lesions of AD and there is a linear correlation between disease activity and the density of $IL\text{-}17^+$ cells [52]. Moreover, IL-17 stimulates keratinocytes to produce VEGF and IL-18. Therefore, it appears that $IL\text{-}17^+$ cells could exaggerate atopic eczema through the release of angiogenic and proinflammatory mediators.

There is evidence that PlGF modulates skin angiogenesis during inflammation and wound healing [53]. Transgenic mice overexpressing PlGF in basal keratinocytes show an increase in the number, branching and size of dermal blood vessels as well as enhanced vascular permeability [54]. PlGF expression is normally very low in the skin, but upregulation has been reported in stimulated keratinocytes [55]. Interestingly, low concentrations of PlGF induce chemotaxis of human mast cells [6].

Thus, different angiogenic factors (VEGFs, Angs, IL-17, etc.) produced by several cellular sources in the inflamed skin, mostly keratinocytes and inflammatory cells (mast cells, macrophages, basophils, eosinophils, Th17 cells, etc.) can contribute to the angiogenic switch in the skin of AD.

Angiogenesis and Lymphangiogenesis in Experimental Models of Atopic Dermatitis

The role of VEGFs in the pathogenesis of AD phenotypes and the effector functions of VEGFs in the skin have not been defined. Even the functional significance of vascular changes of the skin in AD is not altogether clear. Several groups have worked to develop a better understanding of angiogenesis, lymphangiogenesis and vascular remodeling in skin inflammation using animal models.

Angiogenesis is a major pathological feature of a keratin-14 IL-4 transgenic mouse model of AD [56]. This group of investigators showed that in this model of AD, there is a progressive increase in skin tissue mRNA for VEGF-A, but not VEGF-B, -C or -D [42]. Chronic application to the ears of Nc/Nga mice of house dust mite allergens causes skin inflammation resembling certain features of AD. This treatment was associated with VEGF-A overexpression and angiogenesis [57].

Vascular remodeling in ear skin during wound healing has been examined during overexpression of Angs in adult mice [58]. Each Ang evoked different amounts of vascular and lymphatic remodeling at different time periods in wound healing skin tissue. This suggests that each Ang exerts its action somewhat differently on blood and lymphatic remodeling in vivo.

Using a bacterial pathogen-induced model of acute skin inflammation, it has been demonstrated that the lymphangiogenic growth factors (VEGF-C, -D and -A) secreted from macrophages in inflamed skin tissue appear critical not only in lymphatic vessel expansion, but also in antigen clearance and inflammation resolution through enhancement of lymphangiogenesis [59]. The latter observation is interesting because AD patients have increased colonization and superinfection with *Staphylococcus aureus* [30]. However, the possible role of lymphangiogenesis in different phenotypes and phases of AD remains elusive.

Conclusions

Vascular remodeling has been extensively investigated in certain inflammatory skin diseases such as psoriasis. There is some evidence in humans and experimental models of AD that angiogenesis is dysregulated. However, the role of angiogenesis in different forms and phases of AD is not fully understood. The latter concept is of paramount importance because recent insights into the genetic and immunologic mechanisms that drive skin inflammation in AD have led to the discovery that this disorder is more heterogeneous than initially thought. Even more elusive and presumably complex is the role of lymphangiogenesis in skin inflammation. Therefore, it is not surprising that there are still several unanswered questions (table 1).

It is likely that better understanding of altered angiogenesis/lymphangiogenesis in different forms and stages of AD may prove beneficial in the treatment of this

Table 1. Unanswered questions about angiogenesis and lymphangiogenesis in AD

Are angiogenesis and lymphangiogenesis secondary to chronic inflammation and/or reparative processes, or an important early step in AD?
What do other members of the VEGF family (e.g. VEGF-B, -C, -D) besides VEGF-A do in AD?
Could human inflammatory cells, under appropriate circumstances, produce antiangiogenic factors?
What are the precise roles of pro- and antiangiogenic chemokines synthesized by human inflammatory cells in AD?
Several cytokines and chemokines (e.g. IL-8, IL-17) exert proangiogenic effects. What part does IL-17 play in angiogenesis in AD?
Are other angiogenic networks involved in AD (e.g. Angs/Tie receptors, semaphorin/plexin, Delta/Notch)?
VEGFs exert chemotactic effects on human basophils, mast cells, monocytes, etc. Do they have other proinflammatory effects?
What is the importance of lymphangiogenesis in AD? What stimuli drive lymphangiogenesis during skin inflammation?

common inflammatory skin disorder. It is possible that specific inhibitors of various mediators (VEGFs, etc.) and receptors (VEGFRs, Tie-2, etc.) controlling angiogenesis/lymphangiogenesis may offer novel strategies for dealing with treatment of microvascular changes in inflammatory skin disorders. The possible relevance of angiogenesis/lymphangiogenesis in the pathophysiology and therapy of AD makes the study of vascular remodeling in this disorder a priority for future research.

References

1 Carmeliet P, Jain RK: Molecular mechanisms and clinical applications of angiogenesis. Nature 2011; 473:298.

2 Norrmen C, Tammela T, Petrova TV, Alitalo K: Biological basis of therapeutic lymphangiogenesis. Circulation 2011;123:1335.

3 Nguyen A, Hoang V, Laquer V, Kelly KM: Angiogenesis in cutaneous disease: part I. J Am Acad Dermatol 2009;61:921.

4 Staton CA, Valluru M, Hoh L, Reed MW, Brown NJ: Angiopoietin-1, angiopoietin-2 and Tie-2 receptor expression in human dermal wound repair and scarring. Br J Dermatol 2010;163:920.

5 de Paulis A, Prevete N, Fiorentino I, Rossi FW, Staibano S, Montuori N, Ragno P, Longobardi A, Liccardo B, Genovese A, Ribatti D, Walls AF, Marone G: Expression and functions of the vascular endothelial growth factors and their receptors in human basophils. J Immunol 2006;177:7322.

6 Detoraki A, Staiano RI, Granata F, Giannattasio G, Prevete N, de Paulis A, Ribatti D, Genovese A, Triggiani M, Marone G: Vascular endothelial growth factors synthesized by human lung mast cells exert angiogenic effects. J Allergy Clin Immunol 2009;123: 1142.

7 Granata F, Frattini A, Loffredo S, Staiano RI, Petraroli A, Ribatti D, Oslund R, Gelb MH, Lambeau G, Marone G, Triggiani M: Production of vascular endothelial growth factors from human lung macrophages induced by group IIA and group X secreted phospholipases A_2. J Immunol 2010;184:5232.

8 Senger DR, Galli SJ, Dvorak AM, Perruzzi CA, Harvey VS, Dvorak HF: Tumor cells secrete a vascular permeability factor that promotes accumulation of ascites fluid. Science 1983;219:983.

9 De Falco S, Gigante B, Persico MG: Structure and function of placental growth factor. Trends Cardiovasc Med 2002;12:241.

10 Keyt BA, Berleau LT, Nguyen HV, Chen H, Heinsohn H, Vandlen R, Ferrara N: The carboxyl-terminal domain (111–165) of vascular endothelial growth factor is critical for its mitogenic potency. J Biol Chem 1996;271:7788.

11 Maglione D, Guerriero V, Viglietto G, Delli-Bovi P, Persico MG: Isolation of a human placenta cDNA coding for a protein related to the vascular permeability factor. Proc Natl Acad Sci USA 1991;88:9267.

12 Gluzman-Poltorak Z, Cohen T, Herzog Y, Neufeld G: Neuropilin-2 is a receptor for the vascular endothelial growth factor (VEGF) forms VEGF-145 and VEGF-165. J Biol Chem 2000;275:18040.

13 Soker S, Takashima S, Miao HQ, Neufeld G, Klagsbrun M: Neuropilin-1 is expressed by endothelial and tumor cells as an isoform-specific receptor for vascular endothelial growth factor. Cell 1998;92:735.

14 Moyon D, Pardanaud L, Yuan L, Breant C, Eichmann A: Plasticity of endothelial cells during arterial-venous differentiation in the avian embryo. Development 2001;128:3359.

15 Herzog Y, Kalcheim C, Kahane N, Reshef R, Neufeld G: Differential expression of neuropilin-1 and neuropilin-2 in arteries and veins. Mech Dev 2001;109:115.

16 Becker PM, Waltenberger J, Yachechko R, Mirzapoiazova T, Sham JS, Lee CG, Elias JA, Verin AD: Neuropilin-1 regulates vascular endothelial growth factor-mediated endothelial permeability. Circ Res 2005;96:1257.

17 Harfouche R, Hassessian HM, Guo Y, Faivre V, Srikant CB, Yancopoulos GD, Hussain SN: Mechanisms which mediate the antiapoptotic effects of angiopoietin-1 on endothelial cells. Microvasc Res 2002;64:135.

18 Thurston G, Suri C, Smith K, McClain J, Sato TN, Yancopoulos GD, McDonald DM: Leakage-resistant blood vessels in mice transgenically overexpressing angiopoietin-1. Science 1999;286:2511.

19 Zagzag D, Amirnovin R, Greco MA, Yee H, Holash J, Wiegand SJ, Zabski S, Yancopoulos GD, Grumet M: Vascular apoptosis and involution in gliomas precede neovascularization: a novel concept for glioma growth and angiogenesis. Lab Invest 2000;80:837.

20 Tammela T, Saaristo A, Lohela M, Morisada T, Tornberg J, Norrmen C, Oike Y, Pajusola K, Thurston G, Suda T, Yla-Herttuala S, Alitalo K: Angiopoietin-1 promotes lymphatic sprouting and hyperplasia. Blood 2005;105:4642.

21 Fett JW, Strydom DJ, Lobb RR, Alderman EM, Bethune JL, Riordan JF, Vallee BL: Isolation and characterization of angiogenin, an angiogenic protein from human carcinoma cells. Biochemistry 1985;24:5480.

22 Geerts L, Jorens PG, Willems J, De Ley M, Slegers H: Natural inhibitors of neutrophil function in acute respiratory distress syndrome. Crit Care Med 2001;29:1920.

23 Folkman J, Klagsbrun M: Angiogenic factors. Science 1987;235:442.

24 Henke C, Marineili W, Jessurun J, Fox J, Harms D, Peterson M, Chiang L, Doran P: Macrophage production of basic fibroblast growth factor in the fibroproliferative disorder of alveolar fibrosis after lung injury. Am J Pathol 1993;143:1189.

25 Hu DE, Hori Y, Fan TP: Interleukin-8 stimulates angiogenesis in rats. Inflammation 1993;17:135.

26 Brat DJ, Bellail AC, Van Meir EG: The role of interleukin-8 and its receptors in gliomagenesis and tumoral angiogenesis. Neuro Oncol 2005;7:122.

27 Yao Z, Fanslow WC, Seldin MF, Rousseau AM, Painter SL, Comeau MR, Cohen JI, Spriggs MK: Herpesvirus Saimiri encodes a new cytokine, IL-17, which binds to a novel cytokine receptor. Immunity 1995;3:811.

28 Numasaki M, Watanabe M, Suzuki T, Takahashi H, Nakamura A, McAllister F, Hishinuma T, Goto J, Lotze MT, Kolls JK, Sasaki H: IL-17 enhances the net angiogenic activity and in vivo growth of human non-small cell lung cancer in SCID mice through promoting CXCR-2-dependent angiogenesis. J Immunol 2005;175:6177.

29 Takahashi H, Numasaki M, Lotze MT, Sasaki H: Interleukin-17 enhances bFGF-, HGF- and VEGF-induced growth of vascular endothelial cells. Immunol Lett 2005;98:189.

30 Bieber T: Atopic dermatitis. N Engl J Med 2008;358:1483.

31 Leung DY, Bieber T: Atopic dermatitis. Lancet 2003;361:151.

32 Palmer CN, Irvine AD, Terron-Kwiatkowski A, Zhao Y, Liao H, Lee SP, Goudie DR, Sandilands A, Campbell LE, Smith FJ, O'Regan GM, Watson RM, Cecil JE, Bale SJ, Compton JG, DiGiovanna JJ, Fleckman P, Lewis-Jones S, Arseculeratne G, Sergeant A, Munro CS, El Houate B, McElreavey K, Halkjaer LB, Bisgaard H, Mukhopadhyay S, McLean WH: Common loss-of-function variants of the epidermal barrier protein filaggrin are a major predisposing factor for atopic dermatitis. Nat Genet 2006; 38:441.

33 Guttman-Yassky E, Nograles KE, Krueger JG: Contrasting pathogenesis of atopic dermatitis and psoriasis – part I: clinical and pathologic concepts. J Allergy Clin Immunol 2011;127:1110.

34 Guttman-Yassky E, Nograles KE, Krueger JG: Contrasting pathogenesis of atopic dermatitis and psoriasis – part II: immune cell subsets and therapeutic concepts. J Allergy Clin Immunol 2011;127: 1420.

35 Brockow K, Akin C, Huber M, Scott LM, Schwartz LB, Metcalfe DD: Levels of mast-cell growth factors in plasma and in suction skin blister fluid in adults with mastocytosis: correlation with dermal mast-cell numbers and mast-cell tryptase. J Allergy Clin Immunol 2002;109:82.

36 Viac J, Palacio S, Schmitt D, Claudy A: Expression of vascular endothelial growth factor in normal epidermis, epithelial tumors and cultured keratinocytes. Arch Dermatol Res 1997;289:158.

37 Brown LF, Yeo KT, Berse B, Yeo TK, Senger DR, Dvorak HF, van de Water L: Expression of vascular permeability factor (vascular endothelial growth factor) by epidermal keratinocytes during wound healing. J Exp Med 1992;176:1375.

38 Wilgus TA, Matthies AM, Radek KA, Dovi JV, Burns AL, Shankar R, DiPietro LA: Novel function for vascular endothelial growth factor receptor-1 on epidermal keratinocytes. Am J Pathol 2005;167: 1257.

39 Man XY, Yang XH, Cai SQ, Yao YG, Zheng M: Immunolocalization and expression of vascular endothelial growth factor receptors (VEGFRs) and neuropilins (NRPs) on keratinocytes in human epidermis. Mol Med 2006;12:127.

40 Zhang Y, Matsuo H, Morita E: Increased production of vascular endothelial growth factor in the lesions of atopic dermatitis. Arch Dermatol Res 2006;297: 425.

41 Zablotna M, Sobjanek M, Glen J, Niedoszytko M, Wilkowska A, Roszkiewicz J, Nedoszytko B: Association between the –1154 G/A promoter polymorphism of the vascular endothelial growth factor gene and atopic dermatitis. J Eur Acad Dermatol Venereol 2010;24:91.

42 Chen L, Marble DJ, Agha R, Peterson JD, Becker RP, Jin T, Li J, Chan LS: The progression of inflammation parallels the dermal angiogenesis in a keratin 14 IL-4-transgenic model of atopic dermatitis. Microcirculation 2008;15:49.

43 Groneberg DA, Bester C, Grutzkau A, Serowka F, Fischer A, Henz BM, Welker P: Mast cells and vasculature in atopic dermatitis-potential stimulus of neoangiogenesis. Allergy 2005;60:90.

44 Grutzkau A, Kruger-Krasagakes S, Baumeister H, Schwarz C, Kogel H, Welker P, Lippert U, Henz BM, Moller A: Synthesis, storage, and release of vascular endothelial growth factor/vascular permeability factor (VEGF/VPF) by human mast cells: implications for the biological significance of $VEGF_{206}$. Mol Biol Cell 1998;9:875.

45 Marone G, Triggiani M, Genovese A, Paulis AD: Role of human mast cells and basophils in bronchial asthma. Adv Immunol 2005;88:97.

46 Granata F, Staiano RI, Loffredo S, Petraroli A, Genovese A, Marone G, Triggiani M: The role of mast cell-derived secreted phospholipases A_2 in respiratory allergy. Biochimie 2010;92:588.

47 Puxeddu I, Alian A, Piliponsky AM, Ribatti D, Panet A, Levi-Schaffer F: Human peripheral blood eosinophils induce angiogenesis. Int J Biochem Cell Biol 2005;37:628.

48 Augustin HG, Koh GY, Thurston G, Alitalo K: Control of vascular morphogenesis and homeostasis through the angiopoietin-Tie system. Nat Rev Mol Cell Biol 2009;10:165.

49 Miossec P, Korn T, Kuchroo VK: Interleukin-17 and type 17 helper T cells. N Engl J Med 2009;361:888.

50 Numasaki M, Fukushi J, Ono M, Narula SK, Zavodny PJ, Kudo T, Robbins PD, Tahara H, Lotze MT: Interleukin-17 promotes angiogenesis and tumor growth. Blood 2003;101:2620.

51 Honorati MC, Cattini L, Facchini A: IL-17, IL-1β and TNF-α stimulate VEGF production by dedifferentiated chondrocytes. Osteoarthritis Cartilage 2004;12:683.

52 Koga C, Kabashima K, Shiraishi N, Kobayashi M, Tokura Y: Possible pathogenic role of Th17 cells for atopic dermatitis. J Invest Dermatol 2008;128:2625.

53 Odorisio T, Cianfarani F, Failla CM, Zambruno G: The placenta growth factor in skin angiogenesis. J Dermatol Sci 2006;41:11.

54 Odorisio T, Schietroma C, Zaccaria ML, Cianfarani F, Tiveron C, Tatangelo L, Failla CM, Zambruno G: Mice overexpressing placenta growth factor exhibit increased vascularization and vessel permeability. J Cell Sci 2002;115:2559.

55 Failla CM, Odorisio T, Cianfarani F, Schietroma C, Puddu P, Zambruno G: Placenta growth factor is induced in human keratinocytes during wound healing. J Invest Dermatol 2000;115:388.
56 Agha-Majzoub R, Becker RP, Schraufnagel DE, Chan LS: Angiogenesis: the major abnormality of the keratin-14 IL-4 transgenic mouse model of atopic dermatitis. Microcirculation 2005;12:455.
57 Jung MK, Hur DY, Song SB, Park Y, Kim TS, Bang SI, Kim S, Song HK, Park H, Cho DH: Tannic acid and quercetin display a therapeutic effect in atopic dermatitis via suppression of angiogenesis and TARC expression in Nc/Nga mice. J Invest Dermatol 2010;130:1459.
58 Kim KE, Cho CH, Kim HZ, Baluk P, McDonald DM, Koh GY: In vivo actions of angiopoietins on quiescent and remodeling blood and lymphatic vessels in mouse airways and skin. Arterioscler Thromb Vasc Biol 2007;27:564.
59 Kataru RP, Jung K, Jang C, Yang H, Schwendener RA, Baik JE, Han SH, Alitalo K, Koh GY: Critical role of $CD11b^+$ macrophages and VEGF in inflammatory lymphangiogenesis, antigen clearance, and inflammation resolution. Blood 2009;113:5650.

Prof. Dr. Gianni Marone
Department of Clinical Immunology and Allergy, and Center for Basic and Clinical Immunology Research (CISI)
University of Naples Federico II
Via S. Pansini 5
IT–80131 Naples (Italy)
Tel. +39 081 7707492, E-Mail marone@unina.it

Ring J, Darsow U, Behrendt H (eds): New Trends in Allergy and Atopic Eczema.
Chem Immunol Allergy. Basel, Karger, 2012, vol 96, pp 61–72

What Can Dogs Bring to Atopic Dermatitis Research?

Thierry Olivry

Department of Clinical Sciences and Center for Comparative Medicine and Translational Research, College of Veterinary Medicine, North Carolina State University, Raleigh, N.C., USA

Abstract

Besides humans, dogs are the only animals that naturally develop skin lesions of atopic dermatitis (AD). In the last two decades, numerous studies have helped establish the close similarity between human and canine AD at the pathogenesis, clinical, epidemiological and therapeutic levels. The study of dogs with AD could potentially be very useful to human AD research because of the species' historical inbred selection that would permit breed-specific genetic, epidemiological or mechanistic studies. Clinical trials enrolling privately owned dogs are helpful for testing the validity of novel preventive or therapeutic interventions before these are used in human patients. Finally, skin lesions of AD can be provoked via environmental, systemic or epicutaneous allergen challenges in dogs that are spontaneously or experimentally sensitized to common dietary or environmental allergens. These experimental canine AD models have proven their utility to test the efficacy of novel treatment modalities in a preclinical setting. In conclusion, natural or experimental canine AD can provide researchers with a unique model to investigate genetic, epidemiological, mechanistic or treatment facets of the human disease. Due to the unique similarity of the disease in both species, the obtained information would very likely be translatable to human patients.

In humans, atopic dermatitis (AD) is a common chronic pruritic allergic skin disease whose frequency appears to increase in the developed world. Studies on the pathogenesis of AD are limited by the restriction imposed by sample collection in patients – especially children – with this disease. Furthermore, novel treatment modalities for AD normally cannot be tested in human subjects before verification of safety and proof-of-concept studies in animals. To date, the main spontaneous animal model used for studies on the pathogenesis and novel therapeutic strategies of AD has been NC/NgA mice raised in nonspecific pathogen-free conditions [1, 2]. Several other models have been proposed by experimental allergen sensitization or genetic engineering of various mice strains (reviewed in [1]). Even though there are obvious advantages in using relatively inexpensive, easily manipulated mouse models to study this complex human disease, there are obvious limitations in the sometimes very artificial nature of the proposed models and evolutionary distance between rodents and humans that is accompanied by important differences in immunological responses [3]. Furthermore, the size of the animals itself limits side-by-side comparisons of active and control therapeutic experiments, thereby decreasing the advantage of using mouse models in clinical trial design.

For decades, dogs have been known to develop a spontaneous allergic skin disease that has been shown to replicate the characteristics of human AD in many facets. As a result, dogs with AD might represent an ideal 'missing link' for the translation of research discoveries from the laboratory, or from mice, to human patients with this disease.

In this short review, we will discuss key aspects highlighting the similarity between human and canine AD in the hope of triggering additional interest in the 'canine AD model' for the study of this common human skin disease.

Canine Atopic Dermatitis Is a Common Spontaneous Animal Heritable Skin Disease

At this time, canine AD is defined as a genetically predisposed inflammatory and pruritic allergic skin disease with characteristic clinical features associated with IgE antibodies most commonly directed against environmental allergens [4]. It is currently distinguished from 'atopic-like dermatitis', an inflammatory and pruritic skin disease with clinical features identical to those seen in canine AD, but in which an IgE response to environmental or other allergens cannot be documented. In this aspect, the dichotomy of canine AD and atopic-like dermatitis mirrors the separation of human atopic from nonatopic eczema [5].

There is evidence that canine AD is a common disease worldwide. For example, in a survey of more than 30,000 dogs seen by general practitioners in the USA, the diagnosis of AD or allergic skin disease had been made in approximately 9% of the dogs [6]. Similarly, a recent survey of small animal skin diseases in the UK suggested that AD represented nearly 5% of canine dermatoses [7].

There is only one epidemiological study investigating the incidence of AD in the general canine population. In Sweden, examination of pet insurance data suggested that if 1,000 dogs were followed for 1 year, there would be 1.7 new claims for AD during that year [8]. Furthermore, data were provided suggesting that the incidence had risen in the decade preceding this study [8].

The prevalence of AD is likely to have varied over time and geographical locations depending upon the genetic predisposition of popular breeds to develop the disease (reviewed in [9]). There is evidence that canine AD is heritable, at least in golden retrievers and Labradors, which are closely related breeds [10]. At this time, however, a mutation predisposing for the development of canine AD has not been identified. As in humans in which the main AD-predisposing gene [filaggrin (*FLG*)] has mutations that vary depending upon race and geographical locations [11], it is predicted that canine AD is only genetically homogeneous in dogs from the same breed living in the same geographical area [12]. For example, the genomic region harboring the canine *FLG* orthologue was found not to be linked with AD in West Highland white terriers in Australia, the UK and the USA [12–14], while it appears linked to the trait in Labradors in the UK [12].

In summary, in dogs like in humans, AD is a common natural disease that appears to be genetically heterogeneous.

Dogs and Humans with Atopic Dermatitis Exhibit the Same Hypersensitivity Patterns

Dogs with AD most often exhibit IgE hypersensitivity to allergens from the environment, which include house dust and storage mites, pollens, molds and, more rarely, animal epithelia [15]. Such hypersensitivity can be revealed by examining immediate and late-phase reactions after intradermal allergen injections and/or obtaining serum levels of allergen-specific IgE serology [15]. An interesting difference in mite hypersensitivity between human and canine atopic patients is that humans tend to be hypersensitive to low-molecular-weight proteases (e.g. group 1 and 2 allergens) of *Dermatophagoides pteronyssinus*, while dogs will usually develop IgE against high-molecular-weight chitinases of *Dermatophagoides farinae* (i.e. Der f 15, Der f 18) [16, 17].

It is proposed that some, but not all, dogs with AD develop food hypersensitivity that might be present alone or in conjunction with IgE specific for other aeroallergens [18, 19]. Indeed, in a recent international prospective study of 743 dogs with AD that were subjected to a dietary restriction-provocation intervention, food-induced flares of AD were diagnosed in 172 dogs (23%) [20].

Finally, in some dogs with AD, IgE-mediated hypersensitivity can be detected against extracts of *Staphylococcus pseudintermedius* or *Malassezia pachydermatis* [21–23].

At this time, evidence suggesting the existence of IgE autoimmunity in dogs with AD has not been found using skin extracts [24] or keratinocyte cultures (J. Wofford and T. Olivry, unpubl. results, 2009).

In summary, in dogs and humans with AD, there is spontaneous development of IgE against environmental, dietary and microbial allergens, a phenomenon that rarely occurs in mouse AD models.

Canine and Human Atopic Dermatitis Are Phenotypically Similar

In dogs and humans, the diagnosis of AD is mainly clinical: it is made by observation of the presence of pruritus and skin lesions at specific predilection sites [25–27].

Whereas the phenotype of AD is known to evolve with age in human patients [27], changes of phenotypes over time have not yet been studied or documented in dogs with this disease.

In some atopic dogs, there are no visible primary lesions – even in pruritic areas. In most dogs, however, primary lesions of AD consist of erythematous macules, patches and 'micropapules'. Skin lesions seen in dogs with AD are most often secondary, as they reflect chronic self-trauma and skin inflammation, with or without concurrent secondary microbial colonization or infection. Secondary lesions include red-brown 'salivary' staining, excoriations, self-induced alopecia, hyperpigmentation, lichenification and scaling.

The common occurrence of secondary bacterial and/or yeast skin infections might add papules, pustules and crusts, scaling, and greasiness to the characteristic cutaneous lesions.

Whereas transepidermal water loss is increased in both nonlesional and lesional skin of dogs with AD, it is not known if this is accompanied with a subjective feeling of dry skin [28].

As in humans with AD, the 'classical' phenotype of AD is characterized by the presence of the lesions described above on the face and flexural and friction areas. Body regions most commonly affected include the face (especially perilabial and periocular skin), inside aspect of the pinnae, dorsal and ventral interdigital areas, flexural aspects of joints on the extremities (cubital, tarsal, carpal and metatarsal flexures), axillae, abdomen, groin, perineum, and ventral tail (fig. 1). Concurrent otitis externa and auricular pruritus are also commonly seen. Any one, or any combination of the preceding areas can be affected. To complicate the clinical diagnosis, a recent study uncovered breed-to-breed variations in the phenotype of canine AD [29], e.g. flexural dermatitis is seen most often in French bulldogs and Chinese shar-pei while perilabial dermatitis is visible more commonly in Dalmatians and West Highland white terriers [29].

Dogs with AD can be affected with other atopic diseases, such as conjunctivitis, rhinitis and more rarely asthma (especially in experimental models). When dogs have food-induced AD, gastrointestinal signs such as vomiting, soft stools, increased defecation rates or diarrhea are also found in 20–30% of these patients [20, 19].

In summary, the classical phenotype of adult canine AD is very similar to that of humans. Atypical variations are also seen, which could mirror variations in breeds, in genetic determinism and/or the patient's environment.

Canine and Human Atopic Dermatitis Have Similar Treatment Outcome

Recent practice guidelines [30], which incorporated the results of a systematic review of randomized controlled trials [31], established the principles of treatment of acute flares and chronic skin lesions of canine AD. After searching for the cause of flares

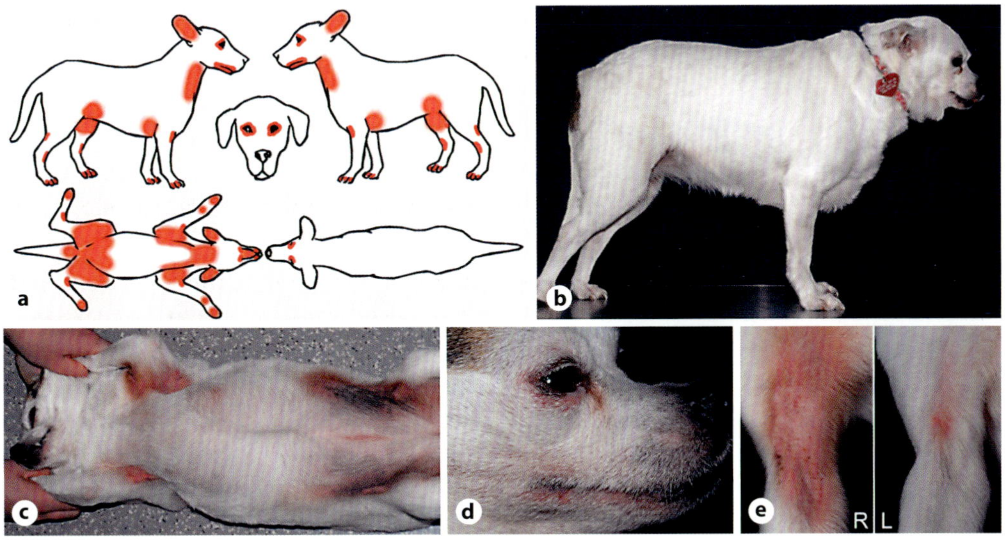

Fig. 1. Canine atopic dermatitis. **a** Diagram showing the distribution of skin lesions (red) in dogs with classical phenotypes. **b–e** Skin lesions in a crossbred dog with AD of classical phenotype. From a distance, lesions can hardly be seen (**b**), but erythema, hyperpigmentation and self-induced alopecia are visible on the axillae, groin (**c**), periocular and perilabial areas (**d**), and flexures of the elbows (**e**; right [R] and left [L]).

(e.g. fleas, food or environmental allergens, skin infections), treatment of acute clinical signs of AD include bathing with nonirritating shampoos and the use of topical or oral glucocorticoids [30, 31]. In addition to glucocorticoids, interventions known to be useful to treat chronic skin lesions of canine AD comprise calcineurin inhibitors (topical tacrolimus, oral cyclosporine) and subcutaneous interferons [30, 31]. As in humans, type 1 histamine receptor antagonists have proven to be of limited clinical benefit [30, 31].

To prevent the recurrence of clinical signs after remission occurs, intradermal allergen injections and allergen-specific IgE serology are performed to select allergens relevant to the pattern of clinical signs for inclusion in subcutaneous allergen-specific immunotherapy [30, 31].

The long-term evolution of canine AD is not known. There is some evidence that, in some dogs with AD (approx. 20%), immunotherapy can be discontinued after 1 year without further recurrence of clinical signs [32], while in most dogs with AD treatment must be continued for years with new hypersensitivities needing to be identified and addressed.

In summary, strategies and interventions aimed at treating clinical signs of canine AD are nearly identical to those of human AD. The outcome of treatment with pharmacological agents is also nearly identical between the two species. Consequently, clinical trials enrolling dogs with AD could be first performed to first determine whether or not a favorable outcome is obtained before the drug is given to human patients with the same disease.

Canine and Human Atopic Dermatitis Have Similar Pathogenesis

For many years, studies on the pathogenesis of canine AD were limited by the availability of canine-specific reagents and small numbers of investigating laboratories. In the last 15 years, however, progress has been made with the study of various facets of the immunopathogenesis of this canine disease; in most cases, results mirror those of studies of human AD. A limitation of most studies, though, is that they usually employed samples from dogs from different breeds that had skin lesions of likely different immunological stages: these factors are a probable source of variability of study results.

Canine AD, like its human counterpart, is not merely a 'type I hypersensitivity reaction'. Subacute and chronic skin lesions have been characterized as a hyperplastic and spongiotic perivascular to diffuse dermatitis rich in mononuclear cells that include lymphocytes and dendritic cells [33]. There is dermal eosinophilia that is often difficult to detect due to eosinophil degranulation [33]. Epidermal Langerhans cells are hyperplastic, often cluster, and express surface IgE [34]. Epitheliotropic lymphocytes in lesional atopic skin possess either αβ or γδ T cell receptors, and they express CD8 more often than CD4 [33]. Mast cell numbers are higher in lesional canine AD than normal canine skin, and they contain and release more histamine after stimulation than normal mast cells [35], which could be due to a higher dermal content of the mast cell stimulator stem cell factor [36].

As in humans, it appears that canine AD skin lesions contain cells transcribing and translating both type 2 and type 1 cytokines, with the latter being present preferentially in chronic lesions [37, 38]. Skin lesions have been shown to be also rich in TNF-α [37–39], stem cell factor [36] and CCL17 (TARC) [40]; the epidermis of canine AD skin also stains positively for thymus stromal lymphopoietin, a prominent Th2 lesion inductor (T. Olivry, unpubl. results).

To date, there are only three published studies on the expression of antimicrobial peptides in the skin of dogs with AD [41]. At this time, there are eight β-defensins (cBD1, cBD2, cBD3, cBD102, cBD103, cBD122 and cBD127) and one cathelicidin (cCath) whose RNA have been shown to be transcribed in canine skin [41–43]. The transcription rate of cBD1 (the hBD1 orthologue) is higher in canine lesional and nonlesional AD skin than in normal canine skin [41]. In contrast, the expression of cBD103 (the hBD3 orthologue) is slightly lower in AD than normal canine skin [41]. Altogether, these results are similar to those seen in human AD skin [44].

As shown for human patients with AD, nonlesional and lesional canine AD skin has a higher rate of colonization and infection with either *S. pseudintermedius* [45] and/or *M. pachydermatis* [46]. As written above, dogs with AD can develop hypersensitivities to microbial allergens, but it is suspected that superantigenic stimulation of immune cells could also contribute to the pathogenesis of AD without the implication of microbial hypersensitivity.

In mammalian skin, the stratum corneum exerts a barrier function that protects from transepidermal water loss and the penetration of exogenous molecules including allergens from the environment. Recently, the new 'outside-inside-outside' theory for the pathogenesis of human AD postulates that a genetic skin barrier defect leads to atopic cutaneous inflammation that further results in decreased SC protein secretion and aggravated barrier dysfunction [47]. At the time of this writing, there is increasing evidence that a skin barrier defect likely exists in dogs with AD (reviewed in [48]). This barrier dysfunction is characterized by abnormal intercellular stratum corneum lipid lamellae, abnormal stratum corneum morphology, reduced and abnormal ceramide content, and (in some but not all dogs) abnormal filaggrin expression. In association with these changes, there is higher transepidermal water loss in atopic than in normal canine skin. Furthermore, atopic inflammation appears to worsen transepidermal water loss and filaggrin expression. It remains unknown, however, if the changes observed are primary (i.e. of genetic origin) or secondary to atopic inflammation that also exists even in clinically normal skin.

In summary, in spite of the markedly lower number of publications investigating the pathogenesis of canine AD compared to those studying the human disease, there is increasing evidence of the strong similarity in the mechanism of these two diseases. This similarity is a strong argument for the appropriateness of canine AD as a model for human AD.

Skin Lesions of Canine (and Human) Atopic Dermatitis Can Be Modeled Experimentally

Intradermal Challenges with Allergens or Anti-IgE Antibodies

As in atopic humans, late-phase reactions (LPR) develop in the skin of atopic dogs after intradermal challenge with allergens to which they are hypersensitive [49, 50]. As normal canine dermal mast cells are naturally covered with IgE [51], similar reactions can be induced in normal and atopic dogs by intradermal injections of anti-canine IgE antibodies that crosslink IgE on high-affinity IgE receptors [50, 52, 53].

Allergen and anti-IgE-induced LPR are macroscopically characterized by erythema, edema and induration [50]. Microscopically, LPR are associated with the sequential migration of neutrophil and eosinophil granulocytes, followed by an infiltration of T lymphocytes and dermal dendritic cells [50, 53]. Such intradermal challenge of normal dogs with anti-IgE antibodies also results in the increased transcription of relevant Th2 cytokines and chemokines [53].

In summary, allergen- and anti-IgE-induced dermal LPR approximate skin lesions of canine AD both macroscopically and microscopically, and they are associated with a cytokine profile similar to that seen in spontaneous disease. While these challenges can be used for rapid testing of antiallergic drugs [54, 55], none of these stimuli produces the epidermal changes seen in naturally occurring AD, thereby limiting the usefulness of IgE-mediated LPR for studying the role of epidermal cells in the development of AD skin lesions.

Epicutaneous Allergen Challenges of Sensitized Dogs
Genetically predisposed dogs can be sensitized to various allergens, including *D. farinae* house dust mites, after repeated weekly epicutaneous applications of allergen extracts [56–58]. In these dogs, allergen-specific peripheral blood T lymphocytes are first activated, followed by an increase in serum allergen-specific IgE levels and cutaneous inflammation at the site of epidermal mite application [56, 57].

The epicutaneous application, via occluded patch tests or painting of allergen extracts on these sensitized dogs results in visible inflammation if elevated serum levels of IgE specific for the challenging allergens are present [56–58]. Inflammation occurs as early as 2 h after provocation, and it increases in severity with time. Microscopic examination of positive tests reveals epidermal microabscesses containing eosinophils, and eosinophil-rich superficial dermal inflammation [56, 58]. Immunohistochemical studies have demonstrated the presence of epidermal Langerhans cell aggregates as well as neighboring clusters of dermal dendritic cells and T lymphocytes in the superficial dermis [56–58]. Forty-eight and 96 h after allergen challenge, the magnitude of the dermal infiltrate correlates with allergen-specific IgE serum levels. Immunoglobulin E-expressing epidermal and dermal dendritic cells are seen in positive patch test reactions [56, 59]. These inflammatory reactions are associated with the concurrent dermal penetration of mite allergens [58]. As for the LPR above, atopy patch tests are associated with the transcription of proallergic cytokines and chemokines [59].

Altogether, results from these studies suggest that epicutaneous applications of relevant allergens, either via painting or occluded patch testing, induce many of the macroscopic, microscopic, and immunological changes seen in spontaneous canine AD skin lesions. As a result, these challenges constitute a relevant model to study mechanisms of atopic skin lesion development [57, 58] or to test the effectiveness and potency of antiallergic drugs [57, 58].

Environmental and Systemic Allergen Challenges of Sensitized Dogs
Dermatophagoides-sensitized beagle dogs experimentally exposed to elevated levels of this allergen in their housing environment develop an erythematous maculopapular dermatitis suggestive of AD [60]. Microscopic examination of lesional skin biopsy specimens reveals early edema and congestion followed by a superficial perivascular-to-diffuse dermatitis rich in mononuclear cells and eosinophils. Epidermal eosinophil exocytosis and abscess formation is seen in late lesions. Immunohistochemical studies further characterize the skin infiltration as including CD4 and CD8-positive

αβ and γδ T lymphocytes as well as dendritic cells; T lymphocytes and dendritic cells are often seen colocalized in dermal and epidermal clusters. Mast cells and dendritic cells express surface IgE [60].

Results from these challenges suggest that this experimental model reproduces most, if not all, of the macroscopic and microscopic changes seen in spontaneously occurring canine AD skin lesions. This model has been used to test the lesion formation potential of various routes of allergen challenge [61], assess the influence of allergen exposure on skin barrier function and morphology [62, 63], and test the effect of antiallergic interventions [64].

Conclusions

In the last two decades, evidence has increased of the profound similarity existing between human and canine AD in the spontaneous development of the disease in young patients, the type and distribution of macroscopic skin lesions, the microscopic changes, and many other aspects of their immunopathogenesis. Furthermore, several experimental models have been developed which provide useful tools to assess the mechanism of skin lesion formation and to rapidly test novel antiallergic interventions.

AD is a complex disease with multiple facets. The existence of a spontaneously arising canine homologue of human AD is unique in that it is common, natural and in a species that shares the same environment as human pet owners. As a result, canine AD is a disease whose study could help advance knowledge important for its human counterpart. It is hoped that the future will see increasing collaborations between medical and veterinary investigators, collaborations that could result in benefit to both human and canine patients.

References

1 Jin H, He R, Oyoshi M, Geha RS: Animal models of atopic dermatitis. J Invest Dermatol 2009;129:31–40.

2 Vestergaard C, Yoneyama H, Matsushima K: The NC/Nga mouse: a model for atopic dermatitis. Mol Med Today 2000;6:209–210.

3 Mestas J, Hughes CC: Of mice and not men: differences between mouse and human immunology. J Immunol 2004;172:2731–2738.

4 Halliwell R: Revised nomenclature for veterinary allergy. Vet Immunol Immunopathol 2006;114: 2007–2008.

5 Johansson SG, Bieber T, Dahl R, Friedmann PS, Lanier BQ, Lockey RF, Motala C, Ortega Martell JA, Platts-Mills TA, Ring J, Thien F, Van Cauwenberge P, Williams HC: Revised nomenclature for allergy for global use: report of the Nomenclature Review Committee of the World Allergy Organization, October 2003. J Allergy Clin Immunol 2004;113: 832–836.

6 Lund EM, Armstrong PJ, Kirk CA, Kolar LM, Klausner JS: Health status and population characteristics of dogs and cats examined at private veterinary practices in the United States. J Am Vet Med Assoc 1999;214:1336–1341.

7 Hill PB, Lo A, Eden CA, Huntley S, Morey V, Ramsey S, Richardson C, Smith DJ, Sutton C, Taylor MD, Thorpe E, Tidmarsh R, Williams V: Survey of the prevalence, diagnosis and treatment of dermatological conditions in small animals in general practice. Vet Rec 2006;158:533–539.

8 Nodtvedt A, Egenvall A, Bergvall K, Hedhammar A: Incidence of and risk factors for atopic dermatitis in a Swedish population of insured dogs. Vet Rec 2006; 159:241–246.

9 Sousa CA, Marsella R: The ACVD task force on canine atopic dermatitis (II): genetic factors. Vet Immunol Immunopathol 2001;81:153–158.

10 Shaw SC, Wood JL, Freeman J, Littlewood JD, Hannant D: Estimation of heritability of atopic dermatitis in Labrador and golden retrievers. Am J Vet Res 2004;65:1014–1020.

11 Akiyama M: FLG mutations in ichthyosis vulgaris and atopic eczema: spectrum of mutations and population genetics. Br J Dermatol 2010;162:472–477.

12 Wood SH, Ollier WE, Nuttall T, McEwan NA, Carter SD: Despite identifying some shared gene associations with human atopic dermatitis the use of multiple dog breeds from various locations limits detection of gene associations in canine atopic dermatitis. Vet Immunol Immunopathol 2010;138:193–197.

13 Barros Roque J, O'Leary CA, Kyaw-Tanner M, Latter M, Mason K, Shipstone M, Vogelnest L, Duffy DL: Haplotype sharing excludes canine orthologous filaggrin locus in atopy in West Highland white Terriers. Anim Genet 2009;40:793–794.

14 Salzman CA, Olivry TJM, Nielsen DM, Paps JS, Harris TL, Olby NJ: Genome-wide linkage study of atopic dermatitis in West Highland White Terriers. BMC Genet 2011;12:37.

15 Hill PB, DeBoer DJ: The ACVD task force on canine atopic dermatitis (IV): environmental allergens. Vet Immunol Immunopathol 2001;81:159–168.

16 McCall C, Hunter S, Stedman K, Weber E, Hillier A, Bozic C, Rivoire B, Olivry T: Characterization and cloning of a major high molecular weight house dust mite allergen (Der f 15) for dogs. Vet Immunol Immunopathol 2001;78:231–247.

17 Weber E, Hunter S, Stedman K, Dreitz S, Olivry T, Hillier A, McCall C: Identification, characterization, and cloning of a complementary DNA encoding a 60-kd house dust mite allergen (Der f 18) for human beings and dogs. J Allergy Clin Immunol 2003;112: 79–86.

18 Olivry T, DeBoer DJ, Prélaud P, Bensignor E: Food for thought: pondering the relationship between canine atopic dermatitis and cutaneous adverse food reactions. Vet Dermatol 2007;18:390.

19 Picco F, Zini E, Nett C, Naegeli C, Bigler B, Rufenacht S, Roosje P, Gutzwiller ME, Wilhelm S, Pfister J, Meng E, Favrot C: A prospective study on canine atopic dermatitis and food-induced allergic dermatitis in Switzerland. Vet Dermatol 2008;19: 150–155.

20 Favrot C, Steffan J, Seewald W, Picco F: A prospective study on the clinical features of chronic canine atopic dermatitis and its diagnosis. Vet Dermatol 2010;21:23–30.

21 Farver K, Morris DO, Shofer F, Esch B: Humoral measurement of type-1 hypersensitivity reactions to a commercial *Malassezia* allergen. Vet Dermatol 2005;16:261–268.

22 Morales CA, Schultz KT, DeBoer DJ: Antistaphylococcal antibodies in dogs with recurrent staphylococcal pyoderma. Vet Immunol Immunopathol 1994;42:137–147.

23 Morris DO, DeBoer DJ: Evaluation of serum obtained from atopic dogs with dermatitis attributable to *Malassezia pachydermatis* for passive transfer of immediate hypersensitivity to that organism. Am J Vet Res 2003;64:262–266.

24 Olivry T, Dunston SM, Pluchino K, Porter K, Hammerberg B: Lack of detection of circulating skin-specific IgE autoantibodies in dogs with moderate or severe atopic dermatitis. Vet Immunol Immunopathol 2008;122:182–187.

25 DeBoer DJ, Hillier A: The ACVD task force on canine atopic dermatitis (XV): fundamental concepts in clinical diagnosis. Vet Immunol Immunopathol 2001;81:271–276.

26 Griffin CE, DeBoer DJ: The ACVD task force on canine atopic dermatitis (XIV): clinical manifestations of canine atopic dermatitis. Vet Immunol Immunopathol 2001;81:255–269.

27 Thestrup-Pedersen K: Clinical aspects of atopic dermatitis. Clin Exp Dermatol 2000;25:535–543.

28 Shimada K, Yoon JS, Yoshihara T, Iwasaki T, Nishifuji K: Increased transepidermal water loss and decreased ceramide content in lesional and non-lesional skin of dogs with atopic dermatitis. Vet Dermatol 2009;20:541–546.

29 Wilhem S, Kovalik M, Favrot C: Breed-associated phenotypes in canine atopic dermatitis. Vet Dermatol 2011;22:143–149.

30 Olivry T, DeBoer DJ, Favrot C, Jackson HA, Mueller RS, Nuttall T, Prélaud P, International Task Force on Canine Atopic Dermatitis: Treatment of canine atopic dermatitis: 2010 clinical practice guidelines from the International Task Force on Canine Atopic Dermatitis. Vet Dermatol 2010;21:233–248.

31 Olivry T, Foster AP, Mueller RS, McEwan NA, Chesney C, Williams HC: Interventions for atopic dermatitis in dogs: a systematic review of randomized controlled trials. Vet Dermatol 2010;21:4–22.

32 Power HT: Why do owners discontinue immunotherapy (abstract). Vet Dermatol 2000;11(suppl 1): 14.

33 Olivry T, Naydan DK, Moore PF: Characterization of the cutaneous inflammatory infiltrate in canine atopic dermatitis. Am J Dermatopathol 1997;19: 477–486.

34 Olivry T, Moore PF, Affolter VK, Naydan DK: Langerhans cell hyperplasia and IgE expression in canine atopic dermatitis. Arch Dermatol Res 1996; 288:579–585.

35 DeMora F, Garcia G, Puigdemont A, Arboix M, Ferrer L: Skin mast cell releasability in dogs with atopic dermatitis. Inflamm Res 1996;45:424–427.

36 Hammerberg B, Olivry T, Orton SM: Skin mast cell histamine release following stem cell factor and high-affinity immunoglobulin E receptor crosslinking in dogs with atopic dermatitis. Vet Dermatol 2001;12:339–346.

37 Nuttall TJ, Knight PA, McAleese SM, Lamb JR, Hill PB: T-helper 1, T-helper 2 and immunosuppressive cytokines in canine atopic dermatitis. Vet Immunol Immunopathol 2002;87:379–384.

38 Olivry T, Dean GA, Tompkins MB, Dow JL, Moore PF: Toward a canine model of atopic dermatitis: amplification of cytokine-gene transcripts in the skin of atopic dogs. Exp Dermatol 1999;8:204–211.

39 Olivry T, Dunston SM, Rivierre C, Jackson HA, Murphy KM, Peters E, Dean GA: A randomized controlled trial of misoprostol monotherapy for canine atopic dermatitis: effects on dermal cellularity and cutaneous tumor necrosis factor-alpha. Vet Dermatol 2003;14:37–46.

40 Maeda S, Tsukui T, Saze K, Masuda K, Ohno K, Tsujimoto H, Iwabuchi S: Production of a monoclonal antibody to canine thymus and activation-regulated chemokine (TARC) and detection of TARC in lesional skin of dogs with atopic dermatitis. Vet Immunol Immunopathol 2005;103:83–92.

41 van Damme CM, Willemse T, van Dijk A, Haagsman HP, Veldhuizen EJ: Altered cutaneous expression of beta-defensins in dogs with atopic dermatitis. Mol Immunol 2009;46:2449–2455.

42 Santoro D, Bunick D, Graves TK, Campbell KL: Expression and distribution of antimicrobial peptides in the skin of healthy beagles. Vet Dermatol 2011;22:61–67.

43 Wingate KV, Torres SM, Silverstein KA, Hendrickson JA, Rutherford MS: Expression of endogenous antimicrobial peptides in normal canine skin. Vet Dermatol 2009;20:19–26.

44 Gambichler T, Skrygan M, Tomi NS, Othlinghaus N, Brockmeyer NH, Altmeyer P, Kreuter A: Differential mRNA expression of antimicrobial peptides and proteins in atopic dermatitis as compared to psoriasis vulgaris and healthy skin. Int Arch Allergy Immunol 2008;147:17–24.

45 Fazakerley J, Nuttall T, Sales D, Schmidt V, Carter SD, Hart CA, McEwan NA: Staphylococcal colonization of mucosal and lesional skin sites in atopic and healthy dogs. Vet Dermatol 2009;20:179–184.

46 White SD, Bourdeau P, Blumstein P, Ibish C, Scott KV, Salman MD, Chapman P: Comparison via cytology and culture of carriage of *Malassezia pachydermatis* in atopic and healthy dogs; in Kwochka KW, Willemse T, VonTscharner C (eds): Advances in Veterinary Dermatology. Oxford, Butterworth-Heinemann 1998, vol 3, pp 292–298.

47 Elias PM, Schmuth M: Abnormal skin barrier in the etiopathogenesis of atopic dermatitis. Curr Opin Allergy Clin Immunol 2009;9:437–446.

48 Olivry T: Is the skin barrier abnormal in dogs with atopic dermatitis? Veterinary Immunology and Immunopathology 2011;144:11–16.

49 Hillier A, Cole LK, Kwochka KW, McCall C: Late-phase reactions to intradermal testing with *Dermatophagoides farinae* in healthy dogs and dogs with house dust mite-induced atopic dermatitis. Am J Vet Res 2002;63:69–73.

50 Olivry T, Murphy KM, Dunston SM, Moore PF: Characterization of the inflammatory infiltrate during IgE-mediated late-phase reactions in the skin of normal and atopic dogs. Vet Dermatol 2001;12:49–58.

51 Halliwell REW: The localization of IgE in canine skin: an immunofluorescent study. J Immunol 1973; 110:422–430.

52 DeBoer DJ, Cooley AJ: Use of induced cutaneous immediate-type hypersensitivity reactions to evaluate anti-inflammatory effects of triamcinolone topical solution in three dogs. Vet Dermatol 2000;11: 25–33.

53 Pucheu-Haston CM, Shuster D, Olivry T, Brianceau P, Lockwood P, McClanahan T, de Waal Malefyt R, Mattson JD, Hammerberg B: A canine model of cutaneous late-phase reactions: prednisolone inhibition of cellular and cytokine responses. Immunology 2006;117:177–187.

54 Bizikova P, Linder KE, Paps JS, Olivry T: Effect of a novel topical diester glucocorticoid spray on immediate and late phase cutaneous allergic reactions in Maltese-Beagle atopic dogs: a placebo-controlled study. Vet Dermatol 2010;21:70–79.

55 Rivierre C, Dunston SM, Olivry T: Effects of a 1 percent hydrocortisone conditioner on the prevention of immediate and late phase reactions in canine skin. Vet Rec 2000;147:739–742.
56 Olivry T, DeAngelo KB, Dunston SM, Clarke KB, McCall CA: Patch testing of experimentally sensitized beagle dogs: development of a model for skin lesions of atopic dermatitis. Vet Dermatol 2006;17: 95–102.
57 Olivry T, Wofford J, Paps JS, Dunston SM: Stratum corneum removal facilitates experimental sensitization to mite allergens in atopic dogs. Vet Dermatol 2011;22:188–196.
58 Pucheu-Haston CM, Jackson HA, Olivry T, Dunston SM, Hammerberg B: Epicutaneous sensitization with *Dermatophagoides farinae* induces generalized allergic dermatitis and elevated mite-specific immunoglobulin E levels in a canine model of atopic dermatitis. Clin Exp Allergy 2008;38:667–679.
59 Marsella R, Olivry T, Maeda S: Cellular and cytokine kinetics after epicutaneous allergen challenge (atopy patch testing) with house dust mites in high-IgE beagles. Vet Dermatol 2006;17:111–120.
60 Marsella R, Olivry T, Nicklin C, Lopez J: Pilot investigation of a model for canine atopic dermatitis: environmental house dust mite challenge of high-IgE-producing beagles, mite hypersensitive dogs with atopic dermatitis and normal dogs. Vet Dermatol 2006;17:24–35.
61 Marsella R, Nicklin C, Lopez J: Studies on the role of routes of allergen exposure in high IgE-producing beagle dogs sensitized to house dust mites. Vet Dermatol 2006;17:306–312.
62 Hightower K, Marsella R, Flynn-Lurie A: Effects of age and allergen exposure on transepidermal water loss in a house dust mite-sensitized beagle model of atopic dermatitis. Vet Dermatol 2010;21:88–95.
63 Marsella R, Samuelson D, Doerr K: Transmission electron microscopic studies in an experimental model of canine atopic dermatitis. Vet Dermatol 2010;21:81–88.
64 Marsella R: Evaluation of *Lactobacillus rhamnosus* strain GG for the prevention of atopic dermatitis in dogs. Am J Vet Res 2009;70:735–740.

Dr. Thierry Olivry
Department of Clinical Sciences, College of Veterinary Medicine, North Carolina State University
1051 Williams Moore Drive
Raleigh, NC 27606 (USA)
Tel. +1 919 513 7711, E-Mail tolivry@ncsu.edu

Ring J, Darsow U, Behrendt H (eds): New Trends in Allergy and Atopic Eczema.
Chem Immunol Allergy. Basel, Karger, 2012, vol 96, pp 73–76

Can Microbial Superantigens Influence Atopic Dermatitis Flares?

Agustin Alomar

Dermatology Department, Institut Universitar Dexeus, Autonomous University of Barcelona, Barcelona, Spain

Abstract

Although atopic dermatitis is accepted as a chronic and recurrent dermatitis, it is clear that several acute flares are due to superficial but not clearly infectious colonization of the skin by bacteria or mold. This short article provides a brief overview of (nearly all) the evidence concerning the possible mechanism of action of this phenomenon.

Atopic dermatitis (AD) is a multifactorial, chronic and relapsing inflammatory skin disease with a genetic predisposition.

Healthy skin is colonized by large numbers of microorganisms. Some bacteria such as coagulase-negative staphylococci (e.g. *Staphylococcus epidermis, Staphylococcus hemolyticus* and *Staphylococcus hominis*) are considered part of the normal skin human flora. These microorganisms are present in proportionally constant numbers in healthy skin. *Staphylococcus aureus* is not considered a member of the normal skin flora [1].

S. aureus skin colonization is found in over 90% of AD patients (in contrast with only 5% of normal individuals) and occurs on both lesional and, to a lesser proportion, nonlesional AD skin [1, 2]. The role of staphylococcal enterotoxins acting as superantigens in AD has recently been recognized and there is now considerable evidence concerning their ability to promote an exacerbation of immune reactivity and allergic skin inflammation in AD.

More than 70% of the *S. aureus* isolated in the skin of AD patients secrete exotoxins such as enterotoxins A, B and C (SEA, SEB and SEC), as well as the toxic shock syndrome toxin 1.

AD skin presents some epidermal alterations which can contribute to an overgrowth of *S. aureus*, such as cutaneous barrier dysfunction, decreased innate immune response (due to low production of cutaneous antimicrobial peptides) and increased proportion of extracellular matrix adhesins for *S. aureus* [1, 3].

Studies suggest that cutaneous colonization by *S. aureus* is 200 times more often in AD skin when compared with healthy skin [1].

Superantigens are viral and bacterial proteins that can specifically induce a polyclonal T lymphocyte activation and stimulate cytokine production [1]. The term superantigen was first introduced by White et al. [4] in 1989 to describe antigens that specifically stimulate the proliferation of T cells in lower concentrations than usual [5]. In addition to T cells, superantigens are also able to cause upregulation of other cell production such as eosinophils, Langerhans cells, macrophages and keratinocytes [5]. Once staphylococcal superantigens penetrate the skin barrier, they contribute to the maintenance and exacerbation of skin inflammation in AD. These staphylococcal exotoxins act as superantigens. Several studies suggest a correlation between the clinical severity of the dermatitis and the colonization by staphylococcal superantigen producers [1, 6–8].

The superantigens are one of the most potent T cell mitogens and can induce the secretion of great amounts of cytokines. Activation and proliferation of T cells induced by superantigens contribute to the exacerbation of AD. In addition, superantigens can increase the proportion of T cells bearing the cutaneous lymphocyte-associated antigen (CLA+), a skin-homing receptor [5, 9].

Other cells such as eosinophils, Langerhans cells, dendritic cells, macrophages and keratinocytes can interact with superantigen inducing the production of proinflammatory cytokines, including IL-1, TNF-α and IL-12 [1, 5].

Effects of *Malassezia* on Immune Response

The possibility of *Malassezia* hypersensitivity in the pathogenesis of AD is suggested in several studies. The high prevalence of type I hypersensitivity to *Malassezia* in AD patients indicates that *Malassezia* antibodies can be important in the pathogenesis of AD [5].

Malassezia yeasts are implicated in AD through production of IgE antibodies that recognize proteins of *Malassezia sympodialis* extract in atopic patients [10]. Positive patch test reactions to *Pityrosporum orbiculare* are described in AD patients [11]. Johansson and colleagues [12] described the correlation of positive patch test reaction to *Malassezia furfur* in vivo with a Th2-like peripheral blood mononuclear response in vitro in AD patients.

Several reports show AD improvement with both topical and systemic antimycotic therapy. Better correlation is verified especially in adults with head-and-neck lesions of AD and seborrheic dermatitis [13–15]. A double-blind, placebo-controlled, randomized study showed that systemic antimycotic therapy decreases the level of specific IgE antibody to *M. furfur*. In contrast, this study does not provide evidence of clinical improvement of systemic antimycotic therapy (ketoconazole) in AD patients [16].

Conclusion

AD is a highly pruritic, multifactorial and chronic skin disease which is genetically determined. The role of superantigens in the pathogenesis of AD flares has been the focus of several studies in the past decade.

Superantigens encompass a family of viral, fungal and bacterial proteins that are able to amplify the immune response in some inflammatory skin diseases such as psoriasis and AD [1, 7]. It has been proven that the presence of staphylococcal superantigens maintains and aggravates the symptoms of AD patients. SEB is the most prevalent superantigen present in AD patients, and applied to normal or atopic skin can induce erythema and dermatitis [1, 7, 8]. Other cells such as eosinophils, Langerhans cells, macrophages and keratinocytes can also interact with bacterial superantigens and modify the course of AD. *Malassezia* spp. are suspected of exacerbating AD disease. The development of specific IgE antibodies and amplification of a Th2 response are probably immune mechanisms related to *Malassezia* colonization on AD skin [10–12].

References

1 Lin YT, Wang CT, Chiang BL: Role of bacterial pathogens in atopic dermatitis. Clinic Rev Allerg Immunol 2007;33:167–177.

2 Williams RE, Gibson AG, Aitchison TC, Lever R, Mackie RM: Assessment of a contact-plate sampling technique and subsequent quantitative bacterial studies in atopic dermatitis. Br J Dermatol 1990;123:493–501.

3 Leung DY, Bieber T: Atopic dermatitis. Lancet 2003;361:151–60.

4 White J, Herman A, Pullen AM, Kubo R, Kappler JW, Marrack P: The V beta-specific superantigen staphylococcal enterotoxin B: stimulation of mature T cells and clonal deletion in neonatal mice. Cell 1989;56:27–35.

5 Baker BS: The role of microorganisms in atopic dermatitis. Clin Exp Immunol 2006;144:1–9.

6 Fukushima H, Hirano T, Shibayama N, et al: The role of immune response to *Staphylococcus aureus* superantigens and disease severity in relation to the sensitivity to tacrolimus in atopic dermatitis. Int Arch Allergy Immunol 2006;141:281–289.

7 Takashi Y, Hideo A, Shigetoshi S, et al: Impaired responses of peripheral blood mononuclear cells to staphylococcal superantigen in patients with severe atopic dermatitis: a role of T cell apoptosis. J Invest Dermatol 2000;8:281–288.

8 Bunikwoski R, Mielke ME, Sharabis H, et al: Evidence for a disease-promoting effect of *Staphylococcus aureus*-derived exotoxins in atopic dermatitis. J Allergy Clin Immunol 2000;105:814–819.

9 Skov L, Baadsgaard O: Bacterial superantigens and inflammatory skin diseases. Clin Exp Dermatol 2000;25:57–61.

10 Johansson S, Karlström K: IgE-binding components in *Pityrosporum orbiculare* identified by an immunoblotting technique. Acta Derm Venereol 1991;71:11–16.

11 Linder MT, Johansson C, Scheynius A: Positive atopic patch test reactions to *Pityrosporum orbiculare* in atopic dermatitis patients. Clin Exp Allergy 2000;30:122–131.

12 Linder MT, Johansson C, Zargari A, et al: Detection of *Pityrosporum orbiculare* reactive T cells from skin and blood in atopic dermatitis and characterization of their cytokines profiles. Clin Exp Allergy 1996;26:1286–1297.

13 Lübbe J: Secondary infections in patients with atopic dermatitis. Am J Clin Dermatol 2003;4:641–654.

14 Bayrou O, Pecquet C, Flahault A, et al: Head and neck atopic dermatitis and malassezia-furfur-specific IgE antibodies. Dermatology 2005;211:107–113.

15 Broberg A, Faergemann J: Topical antimycotic treatment of atopic dermatitis in the head/neck area. Acta Derm Venereol 1995;75:46–49.

16 Bäck O, Bartosik J: Systemic ketoconazol for yeast allergic patients with atopic dermatitis. J Eur Acad Dermatol Venereol 2001;15:34–38.

Further Reading

Bratton DL, May KR, Kailey JM, et al: Staphylococcal toxic shock syndrome toxin-1 inhibits monocyte apoptosis. J Allergy Clin Immunol 2004;103:895–900.

Cardona ID, Cho SH, Leung DYM: Role of bacterial superantigens in atopic dermatitis. Am J Clin Dermatol 2006;7:273–279.

Gallo RL, Murakami M, Ohtake T, Zaiou M: Biology and clinical relevance of naturally occurring antimicrobial peptides. J Allergy Clin Immunol 2002;110:823–831.

Johansson C, Eshaghi H, Tengevall-Linder M, Jakobson E, Scheynius A: Positive atopy patch test reaction to Malassezia furfur in atopic dermatitis correlates with a T helper 2-like peripheral blood mononuclear cells response. J Invest Dermatol 2002;118:1044–1051.

Käagi MK, Joller-Jemelka H, Wüuthrich B: Correlation of eosinophils, eosinophil cationic protein and soluble interleukin-2 receptor with the clinical activity of atopic dermatitis. Dermatology 1992;185:88–92.

Kappler J, Kotzin B, Herron L, et al: V beta-specific stimulation of human T cells by staphylococcal toxins. Science 1989;244:811–813.

Kiehl P, Falkenberg K, Vogelbruch M, Kapp A: Tissue eosinophilia in acute and chronic atopic dermatitis: a morphometric approach using quantitative image analysis of immunostaining. Br J Dermatol 2001;145:720–729.

Kim KH, Han JH, Chung JH, et al: Role of staphylococcal superantigen in atopic dermatitis: influence on keratinocytes. J Korean Med Sci 2006;21:315–323.

Leung DY, Harbeck R, Bina P, Reiser FR, et al: Presence of IgE antibodies to staphylococcal exotoxins onf the skin of patients with atopic dermatitis. Evidence for a new group of allergens. JL Clin Invest 1993;92:1374–1380.

Mangan DF, Robertson B, Wahl SM: IL-4 enhances programmed cell death (apoptosis) in stimulated human monocytes. J Immunol 1992;148:1812–1816.

Morishita Y, Tada J, Sato A, et al: Possible influences of Staphylococcus aureus on atopic dermatitis-the colonizing features and the effects of staphylococcal enterotoxins. Clin Exp Allergy 1999;29:1110–1117.

Ou LS, Goleva E, Hall C, et al: T regulatory cells in atopic dermatitis and subversion of their activity by superantigens. J Allergy Clin Immunol 2004;113:756–763.

Ou LS, Huang JL: Cellular aspects of atopic dermatitis. Clinic Rev Allergy Immunol 2007;33:191–198.

Proft T, Fraser JD: Bacterial superantigens. Clin Exp Immunol 2003;133:299–306.

Schmidt M, Zargari A, Holt P, et al: The complete cDNA sequence and expression of the first major allergenic protein of Malassezia furfur, Mal f 1. Eur J Biochem 1997;246:181–185.

Schroder J-M, Harder J: Human beta-defensin-2. Int J Biochem Cell Biol 1999;31:645–651.

Strange P, Skov L, Lisby S, Nielsen PL, Baadsgaard O: Staphylococcal enterotoxin B applied on intact normal and intact atopic skin induces dermatitis. Arch Dermatol 1996;132:27–33.

Tomai MA, Schlievert PM, Kotb M: Distinct T cell receptor V beta gene usage by human T lymphocytes stimulated with the streptococcal pyrogenic exotoxins and pep M5 protein. Infect Immun 1992;60:701–705.

Wedi B, Wieczorek D, Stunkel T, et al: Staphylococcal exotoxin exert proinflammatory effects through inhibition of eosinophil apoptosis, increased surface antigen expression (CD11b, CD45, CD 54 and CD 69), and enhanced cytokine-activated oxidative burst, thereby triggering allergic inflammatory reaction. J Allergy Clin Immunol 2002;109:477–484.

Zollner TM, Wichellaus TA, Hartung A, et al: Colonization with superantigen-producing Staphylococcus aureus is associated with increased severity of atopic dermatitis. Clin Exp Allergy 2000;30:994–1000.

Prof. Dr. Agustin Alomar
Dermatology Department, Institut Universitar Dexeus, Autonomous University of Barcelona
ES–8028 Barcelona (Spain)
Tel. +34 932150152, E-Mail agustin.alomar@usphospitales.com

Ring J, Darsow U, Behrendt H (eds): New Trends in Allergy and Atopic Eczema.
Chem Immunol Allergy. Basel, Karger, 2012, vol 96, pp 77–80

Inflammation-Induced Alterations in the Skin Barrier Function: Implications in Atopic Dermatitis

Christian Vestergaard[a] · Malene Hvid[b] · Claus Johansen[a] · Kaare Kemp[c] · Bent Deleuran[b] · Mette Deleuran[a]

[a]Department of Dermatology, Aarhus University Hospital, [b]Department of Immunology and Microbiology, Aarhus University, Aarhus, and [c]LEO Pharma, Ballerup, Denmark

Abstract

The pathogenesis of atopic dermatitis (AD) is very complex, but best characterized by an inflammatory reaction in the skin and a disrupted skin barrier. Until recently, these two factors have been studied as separate entities; however, it has been shown that inflammatory cytokines can regulate filaggrin, a very important component of the skin barrier, as well as proteins involved in the processing and maturation of filaggrin. Therefore, inflammation itself may be able to induce a functional skin barrier dysfunction and thereby aggravate the eczematous reaction in AD.

Atopic dermatitis (AD) is a common chronic or chronically relapsing eczematous skin disease. The pathogenesis of this disease has not been completely elucidated, but lately research has focused on two components in the skin: the inflammatory reaction and the skin barrier function.

The inflammatory reaction in the skin has traditionally been described as a Th2-dominated response (i.e. high production of IL-4, IL-5 and IL-13) in the acute phase of the disease and a mixed Th1/Th2 response (i.e. production of IL-2 and IFN-γ in addition) in the chronic phase.

In addition to lymphocytes, inflammatory dendritic cells are also very important in the development of the disease, both as mediators of inflammation and antigen-presenting cells, as well as the keratinocytes that are able to produce chemotactic factors [1].

Thus, a complex network of immune-competent cells and inflammatory factors leads to the inflammation seen in the skin of AD. Very dry skin with increased

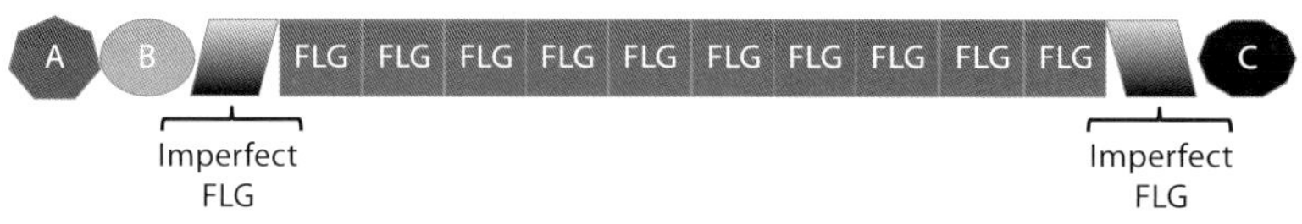

Fig. 1. Schematic representation of the profilaggrin molecule. A and B are the N motifs where A is the S100 calcium-binding motif. This is followed by an imperfect FLG repeat, and thereafter 8–12 filaggrin repeats. The C terminal end consists of an imperfect FLG repeat and a C terminal domain. Modified from Sandilands et al. [4] and McGrath and Uitto [11].

transepidermal water loss (TEWL) is also a prominent feature of AD [2]. Another disease characterized by dry skin and eczema is the genodermatosis ichtyosis vulgaris, and in 2006 the genetic basis for this disease was described as an autosomal recessive trait due to loss-of-function mutations in the FLG gene located on chromosome 1q21 that codes for the (pro)filaggrin molecule [3]. This led to exciting results showing that approximately 30–50% of AD patients are heterozygous for mutations in the FLG gene [4].

Filaggrin is synthesized as a precursor profilaggrin molecule, the structure of which can be seen in figure 1. The regulation of the expression and posttranslational modification of profilaggrin is complex and involves transcription factors AP-1 and p63, phosphorylation by kinases and binding of Ca^{2+} to the N-terminal A motif, which may protect cleavage sites in the molecule through conformational changes. The processing into the active filaggrin molecules involves cleavage of the N-terminal AB-motif, dephosphorylation and proteolysis into free filaggrin molecules. These bind keratin intermediary filaments, and cause aggregation and the condensation of the keratinocytes in the stratum granulosum [4].

Filaggrin has one more role to play though. The breakdown of filaggrin, a process mediated among others by caspase 14, leads to liberation of hygroscopic amino acids that act as natural moisturizing factors (NMF) [5].

Caspase 14, a unique member of the cysteinyl aspartate-specific proteinase family, is expressed primarily in the cornified layers of epithelium such as the epidermis. As mentioned above, caspase 14 has been implicated as an important enzyme in the breakdown of filaggrin into NMF, but it has also been shown that caspase 14 is able to cleave the N-terminal part of profilaggrin. However, experiments with caspase 14 knockout mice show that although the processing of profilaggrin into filaggrin may be altered, filaggrin is still produced in the skin. The breakdown of filaggrin into NMF on the other hand is disturbed, which explains the phenotype of the caspase 14 knockout mice that have increased TEWL, dry skin, hyperlinearity and lichenization. No human equivalent to the caspase 14 knockout has been described [6].

The skin of AD is therefore characterized by an inflammatory reaction in the dermis/epidermis and a decreased skin barrier function in the epidermis. It has been shown that inflammatory cytokines involved in the Th2 response, IL-4 and IL-13, are able to downregulate filaggrin expression and thus induce a functional filaggrin defect, thereby providing a link between inflammation and defective skin barrier function [7, 8]. Additionally, IL-25 (IL-17E), the Th2 response inducer, can downregulate the expression of filaggrin [9].

The expression of filaggrin is not the only skin barrier-related protein that is regulated by inflammatory cytokines. We have shown that caspase 14 expression in keratinocyte cell cultures is downregulated in a dose-dependent manner in response to IL-14, IL-13 and IFN-γ stimulation on both the mRNA and protein levels. Skin biopsies from AD patients have also shown diminished expression of caspase 14 in the stratum granulosum consistent with the results obtained in cell cultures. Yet diminished caspase 14 expression has also been the case in biopsies from contact dermatitis and psoriasis, which is consistent with the results obtained in keratinocyte cell cultures [8]. Skin barrier function is also diminished in patients suffering from contact dermatitis; therefore, an inflammation-induced downregulation of caspase 14 with the subsequent loss of NMF could in part explain the pathogenesis of contact dermatitis. The significance of lower caspase 14 expression in psoriasis skin, however, is unclear.

These results imply that the inflammation may influence the structure of the skin barrier on different levels. Not only does inflammation inhibit filaggrin expression, which inhibits the structural building of the stratum corneum, but also the production of NMF, which may thereby lead to increased TEWL. There is no doubt that filaggrin and mutations in this gene are risk factors for AD. However, a recent observation that TEWL is not significantly higher in AD patients with filaggrin mutations than in AD patients without filaggrin mutations, although both are higher than healthy controls, along with results demonstrating no difference in permeability coefficients between wild-type AD patients and filaggrin mutation patients [10] suggests that, at least this part of the AD phenotype, is dependent on other factors in the skin barrier than filaggrin, and among these could be caspase 14.

References

1 Bieber T: Atopic dermatitis. N Engl J Med 2008;358:1483–1494.

2 Cork MJ, Danby SG, Vasilopoulos Y, Hadgraft J, Lane ME, Moustafa M, et al: Epidermal barrier dysfunction in atopic dermatitis. J Invest Dermatol 2009;129:1892–1908.

3 Palmer CN, Irvine AD, Terron-Kwiatkowski A, Zhao Y, Liao H, Lee SP, et al: Common loss-of-function variants of the epidermal barrier protein filaggrin are a major predisposing factor for atopic dermatitis. Nat Genet 2006;38:441–446.

4 Sandilands A, Sutherland C, Irvine AD, McLean WH: Filaggrin in the frontline: role in skin barrier function and disease. J Cell Sci 2009;122:1285–1294.

5 Denecker G, Ovaere P, Vandenabeele P, Declercq W: Caspase-14 reveals its secrets. J Cell Biol 2008;180:451–458.
6 Denecker G, Hoste E, Gilbert B, Hochepied T, Ovaere P, Lippens S, et al: Caspase-14 protects against epidermal UVB photodamage and water loss. Nat Cell Biol 2007;9:666–674.
7 Howell MD, Kim BE, Gao P, Grant AV, Boguniewicz M, Debenedetto A, et al: Cytokine modulation of atopic dermatitis filaggrin skin expression. J Allergy Clin Immunol 2007;120:150–155.
8 Hvid M, Johansen C, Deleuran B, Kemp K, Deleuran M, Vestergaard C: Regulation of caspase 14 expression in keratinocytes by inflammatory cytokines – a possible link between reduced skin barrier function and inflammation? Exp Dermatol 2011;20:633–636.
9 Hvid M, Vestergaard C, Kemp K, Christensen GB, Deleuran B, Deleuran M: IL-25 in atopic dermatitis: a possible link between inflammation and skin barrier dysfunction? J Invest Dermatol 2011;131:150–157.
10 Jakasa I, Koster ES, Calkoen F, McLean WH, Campbell LE, Bos JD, et al: Skin barrier function in healthy subjects and patients with atopic dermatitis in relation to filaggrin loss-of-function mutations. J Invest Dermatol 2011;131:540–542.
11 McGrath JA, Uitto J: The filaggrin story: novel insights into skin-barrier function and disease. Trends Mol Med 2008;14:20–27.

Dr. Christian Vestergaard
Department of Dermatology, Aarhus University Hospital
P.P. Ørums Gade 11
DK–8000 Aarhus C (Denmark)
Tel. +45 8949 1861, E-Mail chrivest@rm.dk

Ring J, Darsow U, Behrendt H (eds): New Trends in Allergy and Atopic Eczema.
Chem Immunol Allergy. Basel, Karger, 2012, vol 96, pp 81–88

Itch and Eczema

Ulf Darsow[a,b,d] · Florian Pfab[a,b,d] · Michael Valet[c] · Thomas R. Tölle[c] · Johannes Ring[a,d]

[a]Klinik und Poliklinik für Dermatologie und Allergologie am Biederstein, [b]KKG Helmholtz Zentrum, [c]Klinik für Neurologie, Klinikum rechts der Isar, Technisches Universität München, and [d]Christine Kühne Center for Allergy Research and Education (CK-CARE), Munich, Germany

Abstract

Eczema/dermatitis belongs to the most pruritic of skin diseases. Pruritogenic mediators in the skin are still mostly unknown. Recent studies, however, have shown that the histamine 4 receptor plays an important role in itch pathophysiology; tryptase and IL-31 are also involved in atopic eczema itch. Differences in itch perception and itch kinetics between healthy volunteers and eczema patients point towards ongoing central nervous inhibitory activity in patients. Questionnaire studies reported comparatively higher loads in affective items chosen by patients with atopic eczema. In the concept of eczema patient management, the therapy of clinical pruritus has to consider pathophysiology and perception by combining topical and systemic treatment.

Itch is one of the most important symptoms in inflammatory skin diseases and allergic disorders. For centuries, it has been defined as an 'unpleasant sensation, eliciting the urge to scratch' [1]. Moreover, itch is an essential diagnostic feature of atopic eczema [eczema, atopic dermatitis (AD)], in association with the markedly better characterized criteria: age-related eczematous appearance and localization, history and clinical signs of atopy, and IgE-mediated sensitization [2].

Pathophysiology

A specific chemosensitive subpopulation of C-fibers has been described as mediating histamine-induced itch [3–5]. Today, this specific pathway for itch is seen as part of a network, which also involves unspecific afferents, adding information on the context of skin inflammation [6]. A role for mast cell tryptase and its receptor on nociceptive afferents (PAR-2) in atopic itch has been proposed because enhanced immunostaining for PAR-2 was found in lesional skin of patients with AD [7]. The neuroimmunological

Table 1. Features of itch in atopic eczema: summary of questionnaire studies

Sensation: sharp, stinging, burning, tickling, pricking [21, 26]
Quality of life: high emotional burden [21, 26, 27]
Frequency: 28% daily, only in 11% of patients was there no itch for more than 1 month [27]
Frequency (Web questionnaire): 91% daily [26]
Intensity: VAS mean 62-79±23%, peak evening and night [21, 27]
Classification: acute itch with atopic eczema lesions vs. chronic itch [27]
Therapy: often no response to antihistamines [27]

interactions between allergen-specific inflammation and sensory nervous system are still under investigation [8, 9]. There is evidence that products of sensory nerves (neuropeptides) can modulate antigen presentation, inflammation and itch in the skin.

Histamine is the most important known itch mediator and was found to be increased in AD lesions [10, 11]. However, the histamine 1(H1) receptor is unlikely to play a major role in AD because the clinical efficacy of nonsedating antihistamines in this disease is very limited [12]. Recent studies have shown that the H4 receptor plays an important role in itch pathophysiology in AD patients [13, 14]. Activation of H4 receptors on Th2 cells increases the production of IL-31 [14]. This cytokine is supposed to be another important itch inducer in AD [15]. To date, no H4 or IL-31 antagonists are available for the treatment of AD itch. Other mediators of atopic itch in the skin are still mostly enigmatic, although many candidates have been investigated and characterized [8, 16–18].

Alloknesis, a phenomenon involving the central projection neurons of the itch afferents [19], plays an important role in the irritability of atopic skin: a certain area of clinically noninvolved skin surrounding an itching lesion may be perceived as itching after slight mechanical stimulation like contact with wool fibers [19].

Itch Questionnaires in Atopic Eczema

The peculiarities of pruritus in AD have been investigated by different groups with different questionnaire instruments but consistent results (table 1). We developed a multidimensional questionnaire, the Eppendorf Itch Questionnaire (EIQ) [20, 21], designed in analogy to the established McGill Pain Questionnaire [22] in pain research. The EIQ was used in therapy assessment and evaluated in an atopy patch test model for AD [23]. The German version of this questionnaire was used in 108 patients with acute AD in comparison to the SCORAD severity index [21]. A principal component analysis with varimax rotation identified main factors of clinical itch. It was shown that atopic itch is a multidimensional sensation with 12 clusters of descriptors, but on a more general level, descriptors could be integrated in three main components (explaining 58% of total variance) which describe the atopic itch. Component A, 'suffering', described the decrease in quality of life caused by pruritus. Main component B contained the quality of the sensation itself (wave-formed and prickling, as well as further descriptors). Component C was a compulsive component describing loss of control and warm feelings. Surprisingly, this component comprised also positive emotional descriptors which were chosen by the patients, and it was the only main component that was not significantly related to the eczema severity (SCORAD). Component C may represent an important factor of the so-called 'itch-scratch cycle' in AD. Comparing the itch sensation of patients with chronic urticaria and AD with visual analogue scales and the EIQ, we found that the difference between these diseases is not a function of pure itch intensity itself, but of the differentiated perception of the symptom: the mean total EIQ score in patients with AD was markedly higher. This was mainly due to higher loads in affective items chosen by patients with AD. It may be speculated that this phenomenon is a feature of chronification of the itch sensation.

The results of these studies show that clinical itch can only partially be quantified by visual analogue scales [24]. The sensation of itch needs an increasing number of descriptors with higher intensities [25]. These descriptors correlate in a complex manner with objective parameters of skin inflammation in AD [21]. Like pain, the subjective perception of itch is an emotional experience with individual thresholds of sensation. Quantity and quality of the sensations are influenced by each other [25]. Thus, central nervous components contribute significantly to the clinical symptom.

All recent questionnaire studies consistently showed a high emotional burden and high chronicity as features of AD itch [21, 26, 27] (table 1).

Processing of the Itch Sensation in the Human Brain

Volunteer Studies

The first studies to investigate the effect of histamine-induced itch correlated subjective itch sensation with central activation using positron emission tomography (PET) as in pain studies [28–30]. A new approach using thermal modulation of histamine-induced itch [31] now also enables functional (fMRI) studies on itch [32, 33]: the cerebral activation pattern of itch processing in 12 healthy volunteers with functional MRI [33] could be investigated, and showed that the changes during the first 8 s of itch induction were reflected by the highest brain modulation (fig. 1). Activated regions were the thalamus, pre-SMA, lateral prefrontal cortex, anterior insular cortex and inferior parietal cortex, whereas the medial frontal cortex, the orbitofrontal cortex, the dorsal part of the anterior cingulate cortex and the primary motor cortex (M1) were less active during histamine-induced itch than during a saline control stimulus. Table 2 gives an overview on the functions of identified regions of interest.

Mochizuki et al. [34] directly compared itch and pain stimuli with fMRI in healthy volunteers. Neural activation in the posterior cingulate cortex and the posterior insula was significantly higher during itch than during pain; pain in contrast to itch induced an activation of the thalamus correlating to subjective pain sensation.

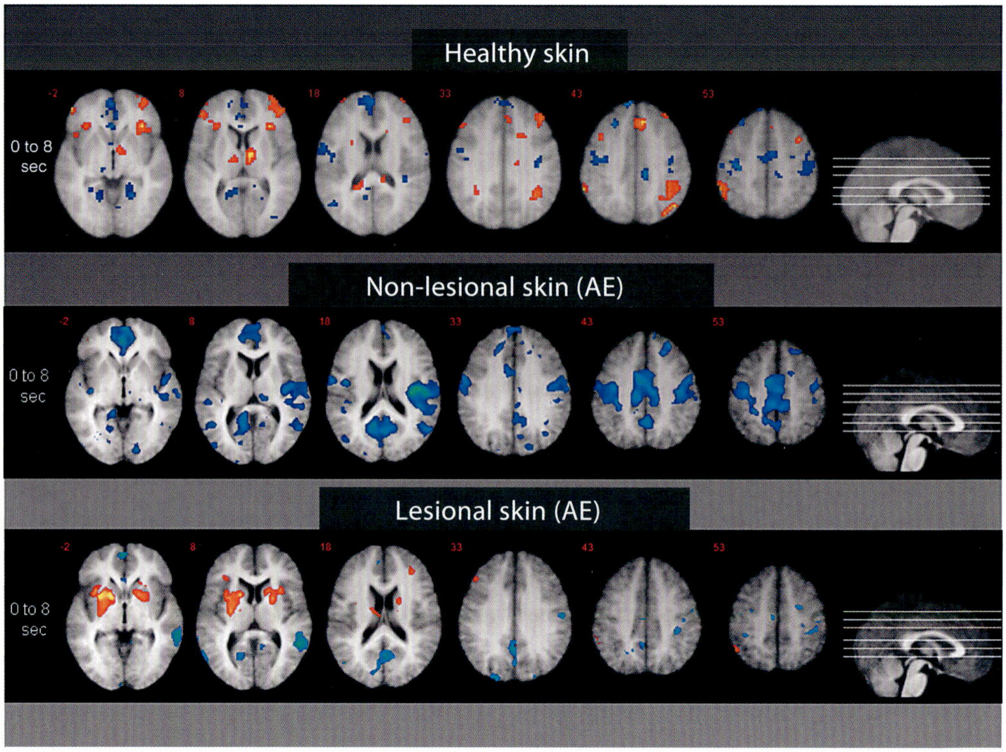

Fig. 1. Cerebral activation pattern of histamine-induced itch in healthy skin of volunteers compared to nonlesional skin of patients with atopic eczema (AE) and lesional skin of these patients during the early (here: first 8 s) phase of itch induction. Blue: deactivation; red: activation [32]. In nonlesional skin of AD patients, fMRI revealed a cerebral deactivation pattern in itch processing structures (thalamus, prefrontal, cingulate, insular, somatosensory and motor cortex) at the beginning of the itch provocation. In contrast, lesional skin showed an activation instead of deactivation pattern already at the beginning of the stimulation in the above-mentioned structures.

In contrast to the aforementioned studies investigating the neuronal effects of pruritus, a recently published fMRI study focused on another aspect, namely scratching [35]. However, a limitation of this study might be that sensory effects of scratching without any induction of itch were measured.

So far, only two studies have used a stimulus method that achieved strong repeatable pruritus comparing itch and non-itch periods within seconds [33] or minutes [36].

Patient Studies

In patients with AD, the initial phase of itch in nonlesional skin produced a cerebral deactivation pattern in itch-processing structures (thalamus, prefrontal, cingulate, insular, somatosensory and motor cortex) on fMRI (fig. 1) [32]. During the course of stimulation, cerebral deactivation was reduced with time and activation of the basal

Table 2. Experimental itch: significantly activated regions and functions (numbers) in the central nervous system as characterized by PET and fMRI studies [32, 50]

(1) Pre-SMA, motor cortex, motor part of cingulum: motor planning, imagination and execution; deactivation shows suppression in volunteers not allowed to scratch	
(2) Thalamus and primary somatosensory cortex: sensory processing, localization, discrimination, detection and intensity encoding of sensory stimuli	
(2, 3) Insula/cingulum: subjective feeling, integration of sensory und emotional experience; interoceptive system	
(4) Inferior parietal and dorsolateral prefrontal cortex: body scheme, integration of multisensory information of all areas relevant for itch; cognitive, evaluative, executing functions	
(2) Sensory (what-where intensity?)	(3) Emotional (how unpleasant?)
(4) Cognitive (circumstances?)	(1) Countermeasures

ganglia occurred instead. In contrast, stimulation in lesional skin resulted in activation instead of deactivation patterns already at the beginning of the stimulation in the above-mentioned structures (fig. 1, table 2).

The differences in itch perception and itch kinetics between healthy volunteers and nonlesional skin in patients point towards ongoing central inhibitory activity in patients with AD, especially at the beginning of the itch provocation.

Another study investigated the effect of allergen-induced itch in patients with mucosal atopy showing similarities to histamine-itch [37].

Therapy of Itch in Eczema

Unfortunately, to date, only a few specific treatment modalities for itch are available. Considering the extensive activation of cortex areas in the human brain in experimental histamine itch models in patients with AD (see above), peripheral and central nervous components can probably be modulated independently. Thus, the therapy of clinical eczema pruritus has to consider both sides of origin and perception of itch, namely the skin and the central nervous system. In clinical practice, intensive pruritus can also exist with nonextensive skin lesions. In younger children, the situation may be more difficult since no clear descriptions of the itch can be obtained. Avoidance of specific and unspecific trigger factors and appropriate basic therapy with emollients are the mainstay of antipruritic therapy in AD [38]. In general, acute itch can be successfully treated with the control of skin inflammation with topical corticosteroids. Limited efficacy of sedating antihistamines (clinical routine) and opioid antagonists (nalmefene, experimental) in atopic itch is known [39]. Table 3 summarizes antipruritic therapies according to the actual EDF guidelines on AD treatment [38]. Use of sedating antihistamines like doxylamine succinate, dimethindene maleate, clemastine or hydroxyzine should be

Table 3. Therapy of itch in atopic eczema

Therapeutic modalities	Examples
General principles	emollients/basis therapy to reduce dry skin; elimination of provocative factors: avoidance of too long and hot bathing, contact with irritant substances or allergens
Experimental physical modalities	acupuncture; cutaneous field stimulation
Anti-inflammatory therapy	corticosteroids (t[1]); ciclosporine (o[1]); tacrolimus (t[1]); Pimecrolimus (t[1]); Ultraviolet light (NB-UVB)
Adjuvant specific antipruritic therapies	creams/lotions containing urea, camphor, menthol, polidocanol or N-palmitoylethanolamide (t); capsaicin (t); opioid receptor antagonists (o[1]; e.g. naltrexone)
Sedation	sedative antihistamines (o)

t = Topically; o = orally.
[1] Evidence-based effect on pruritus as proven by randomized controlled studies.

limited to phases of acute exacerbations, and is increasingly becoming controversial. Administration in the evenings is recommended. In 10–15% of children, paradoxical side effects were described (hyperactivity). The role of nonsedating antihistamines for treatment of atopic itch is also under discussion due to limited therapeutic effects [40]. An evidence-based review of studies on the efficacy of antihistamines in the treatment of AD itch was published by Klein and Clark [41]. Further studies on this topic are necessary. Additional H2 antihistamines seem to be of no additional clinical value [42]. Regarding experimental histamine-induced as well as allergen-induced itch, acupuncture showed promising effects in healthy volunteers [43–46] and patients with AD [47]. Again, further clinical studies with this treatment are necessary.

Some topical compounds which are used in adults as antipruritics (e.g. phenol and menthol) may be toxic or irritative in children. Topical treatment with antihistamines or anesthetics is not recommended, due to a possible sensitizing potential. The tricyclic antiwdepressant doxepin is topically used for the relief of itch in AD from 12 years on, but contact dermatitis may develop [48]. In addition, the treated skin area is limited to 10% to avoid central nervous side effects due to absorption. Best results are obtained when combined strategies which are dermatologically adequate for the underlying disease are used. For eczema, this means a concept of patient management [49] including rehydrating emollient baseline therapy and appropriate on-demand anti-inflammatory treatment with topical steroids, allergy diagnosis [2] and, in selected cases, topical or systemic immunosuppressants, antibiotics or phototherapy, and modification of scratch behavior by patient counseling [38]. The impact of pruritus on the quality of life of patients should not be underestimated.

References

1 Hafenreffer S: De pruritu; in Kühnen B (ed): Nosodochium, in quo cutis, eique adaerentium partium, affectus omnes, singulari methodo, et cognoscendi et curandi fidelissime traduntur. Ulm 1660, pp 98–102.

2 Ring J: Allergy in Practice. Berlin, Springer, 2005.

3 Schmelz M: A neural pathway for itch. Nat Neurosci 2001;4:9–10.

4 Schmelz M, Hilliges M, Schmidt R, Orstavik K, Vahlquist C, Weidner C, et al: Active 'itch fibers' in chronic pruritus. Neurology 2003;61:564–566.

5 Schmelz M, Schmidt R, Bickel A, Handwerker HO, Torebjörk HE: Specific C-receptors for itch in human skin. J Neurosci 1997;17:8003–8008.

6 Schmelz M: Itch and pain. Neurosci Biobehav Rev 2010;34:171–176.

7 Steinhoff M, Neisius U, Ikoma A, Fartasch M, Heyer G, Skov PS, et al: Proteinase-activated receptor-2 mediates itch: a novel pathway for pruritus in human skin. J Neurosci 2003;23:6176–6180.

8 Steinhoff M, Bienenstock J, Schmelz M, Maurer M, Wei E, Biro T: Neurophysiological, neuroimmunological, and neuroendocrine basis of pruritus. J Invest Dermatol 2006;126:1705–1718.

9 Buddenkotte J, Steinhoff M: Pathophysiology and therapy of pruritus in allergic and atopic diseases. Allergy 2010;65:805–821.

10 Johnson HH, DeOreo GA, Lascheid WP, Mitchell F: Skin histamine levels in chronic atopic dermatitis. J Invest Dermatol 1960;34:237–238.

11 Juhlin L: Localization and content of histamine in normal and diseased skin. Acta Derm Venereol 1967;47:383–391.

12 Wahlgren CF, Hägermark Ö, Bergström R: The antipruritic effect of a sedative and a non-sedative antihistamine in atopic dermatitis. Br J Dermatol 1990; 122:545–551.

13 Dijkstra D, Leurs R, Chazot P, Shenton FC, Stark H, Werfel T, et al: Histamine downregulates monocyte CCL2 production through the histamine H4 receptor. J Allergy Clin Immunol 2007;120:300–307.

14 Gutzmer R, Mommert S, Gschwandtner M, Zwingmann K, Stark H, Werfel T: The histamine H4 receptor is functionally expressed on Th2 cells. J Allergy Clin Immunol 2009;123:619–625.

15 Sonkoly E, Muller A, Lauerma AI, et al: IL-31: a new link between T cells and pruritus in atopic skin inflammation. J Allergy Clin Immunol 2006;117: 411–417.

16 Darsow U, Scharein E, Bromm B, Ring J: Skin testing of the pruritogenic activity of histamine and cytokines (interleukin-2 and tumour necrosis factor-alpha) at the dermal-epidermal junction. Br J Dermatol 1997;137:415–417.

17 Ständer S, Steinhoff M, Schmelz M, Weisshaar E, Metze D, Luger T: Neurophysiology of pruritus: cutaneous elicitation of itch. Arch Dermatol 2003;139: 1463–1470.

18 Ständer S, Weisshaar E, Luger TA: Neurophysiological and neurochemical basis of modern pruritus treatment. Exp Dermatol 2008;17:161–169.

19 Heyer G, Ulmer FJ, Schmitz J, Handwerker HO: Histamine-induced itch and alloknesis (itchy skin) in atopic eczema patients and controls. Acta Derm Venereol 1995;75:348–352.

20 Darsow U, Mautner VF, Bromm B, Scharein E, Ring J: The Eppendorf Pruritus Questionnaire (in German). Hautarzt 1997;48:730–733.

21 Darsow U, Scharein E, Simon D, Walter G, Bromm B, Ring J: New aspects of itch pathophysiology: component analysis of atopic itch using the 'Eppendorf Itch Questionnaire'. Int Arch Allergy Immunol 2001;124:326–331.

22 Melzack R: The McGill Pain Questionnaire: major properties and scoring methods. Pain 1975;1:277–299.

23 Weissenbacher S, Bacon T, Targett D, Behrendt H, Ring J, Darsow U: Atopy patch test-reproducibility and elicitation of itch in different application sites. Acta Derm Venereol 2005;85:147–151.

24 Hägermark O, Wahlgren CF: Some methods for evaluating clinical itch and their application for studying pathophysiological mechanisms. J Dermatol Sci 1992;4:55–62.

25 Darsow U, Ring J, Scharein E, Bromm B: Correlations between histamine-induced wheal, flare and itch. Arch Dermatol Res 1996;288:436–441.

26 Dawn A, Papoiu AD, Chan YH, Rapp SR, Rassette N, Yosipovitch G: Itch characteristics in atopic dermatitis: results of a web-based questionnaire. Br J Dermatol 2009;160:642–644.

27 Chrostowska-Plak D, Salomon J, Reich A, Szepietowski JC: Clinical aspects of itch in adult atopic dermatitis patients. Acta Derm Venereol 2009;89:379–383.

28 Darsow U, Drzezga A, Frisch M, Munz F, Weilke F, Bartenstein P, et al: Processing of histamine-induced itch in the human cerebral cortex: a correlation analysis with dermal reactions. J Invest Dermatol 2000;115:1029–1033.

29 Hsieh JC, Hägermark O, Stahle-Backdahl M, Ericson K, Eriksson L, Stone-Elander S, et al: Urge to scratch represented in the human cerebral cortex during itch. J Neurophysiol 1994;72:3004–3008.
30 Hsieh JC, Meyerson BA, Ingvar M: PET study on central processing of pain in trigeminal neuropathy. Eur J Pain 1999;3:51–65.
31 Pfab F, Valet M, Sprenger T, Tölle TR, Athanasiadis GI, Behrendt H, et al: Short-term alternating temperature enhances histamine-induced itch: a biphasic stimulus model. J Invest Dermatol 2006;126: 2673–2678.
32 Pfab F, Valet M, Sprenger T, Huss-Marp J, Athanasiadis GI, Baurecht HJ, Konstantinow A, Zimmer C, Behrendt H, Ring J, Tölle TR, Darsow U: Temperature modulated histamine-itch in lesional and nonlesional skin in atopic eczema – a combined psychophysical and neuroimaging study. Allergy 2010;65:84–94.
33 Valet M, Pfab F, Sprenger T, Woller A, Zimmer C, Behrendt H, et al: Cerebral processing of histamine-induced itch using short-term alternating temperature modulation – an fMRI study. J Invest Dermatol 2008;128:426–433.
34 Mochizuki H, Sadato N, Saito DN, Toyoda H, Tashiro M, Okamura N, et al: Neural correlates of perceptual difference between itching and pain: a human fMRI study. Neuroimage 2007;36:706–717.
35 Yosipovitch G, Ishiuji Y, Patel TS, Hicks MI, Oshiro Y, Kraft RA, et al: The brain processing of scratching. J Invest Dermatol 2008;128:1806–1811.
36 Herde L, Forster C, Strupf M, Handwerker HO: Itch induced by a novel method leads to limbic deactivations a functional MRI study. J Neurophysiol 2007; 98:2347–2356
37 Leknes SG, Bantick S, Willis CM, Wilkinson JD, Wise RG, Tracey I: Itch and motivation to scratch: an investigation of the central and peripheral correlates of allergen- and histamine-induced itch in humans. J Neurophysiol 2007;97:415–422.
38 Ring J, Alomar A, Bieber T, Deleuran M, Fink-Wagner A, Gelmetti C, Gieler G, Lipozencic J, Luger T, Oranje AP, Schäfer T, Schwennesen T, Seidenari S, Simon D, Ständer S, Stingl G, Szalai S, Szepietowski JC, Taïeb A, Werfel T, Wollenberg A, Darsow U: Guidelines for treatment of atopic eczema (atopic dermatitis). J Eur Acad Derm Venereol 2011, submitted.
39 Monroe EW: Efficacy and safety of nalmefene in patients with severe pruritus caused by chronic urticaria and atopic dermatitis. J Am Acad Dermatol 1989;21:135–136.
40 Ständer S, Weisshaar E, Mettang T, Szepietowski JC, Carstens E, Ikoma A, et al: Clinical classification of itch: a position paper of the International Forum for the Study of Itch. Acta Derm Venereol 2007;87:291–294.
41 Klein PA, Clark RA: An evidence-based review of the efficacy of antihistamines in relieving pruritus in atopic dermatitis. Arch Dermatol 1999;135:1522–1525.
42 Foulds IS, MacKie RM: A double-blind trial of the H2 receptor antagonist cimetidine, and the H1 receptor antagonist promethazine hydrochloride in the treatment of atopic dermatitis. Clin Allergy 1981;11:319–323.
43 Pfab F, Hammes M, Backer M, Huss-Marp J, Athanasiadis GI, Tölle TR, et al: Preventive effect of acupuncture on histamine-induced itch: a blinded, randomized, placebo-controlled, crossover trial. J Allergy Clin Immunol 2005;116:1386–1388.
44 Belgrade MJ, Solomon LM, Lichter EA: Effect of acupuncture on experimentally induced itch. Acta Derm Venereol 1984;64:129–133.
45 Lundeberg T, Bondesson L, Thomas M: Effect of acupuncture on experimentally induced itch. Br J Dermatol 1987;117:771–777.
46 Kesting MR, Thurmuller P, Holzle F, Wolff KD, Holland-Letz T, Stucker M: Electrical ear acupuncture reduces histamine-induced itch (alloknesis). Acta Derm Venereol 2006;86:399–403.
47 Pfab F, Huss-Marp J, Gatti A, Fuqin J, Athanasiadis GI, Irnich D, Raap U, Schober W, Behrendt H, Ring J, Darsow U: Influence of acupuncture on type I hypersensitivity itch and the wheal and flare response in adults with atopic eczema – a blinded, randomized, placebo-controlled, crossover trial. Allergy 2010;65:903–910.
48 Doxepin cream for eczema? Drug Ther Bull 2000; 38:31–32.
49 Ring J, Brockow K, Abeck D: The therapeutic concept of 'patient management' in atopic eczema. Allergy 1996;51:206–215.
50 Pfab F, Valet M, Tölle T, Behrendt H, Ring J, Darsow U: Recent progress in unraveling central nervous processing of itch sensation. WAO J 2008;1:168–173.

Prof. Dr. med. Ulf Darsow
Klinik und Poliklinik für Dermatologie und Allergologie am Biederstein, Technische Universität München
Biedersteiner Strasse 29
DE–80802 Munich (Germany)
Tel. +49 89 4140 3170, E-Mail ulf.darsow@lrz.tum.de

Ring J, Darsow U, Behrendt H (eds): New Trends in Allergy and Atopic Eczema.
Chem Immunol Allergy. Basel, Karger, 2012, vol 96, pp 89–95

Eczema Herpeticum

Andreas Wollenberg

Department of Dermatology, Ludwig Maximilian University, Munich, Germany

Abstract

Atopic dermatitis (AD) patients tend to develop viral infections such as herpes simplex, molluscum contagiosum or verrucae vulgares more frequently than nonatopic patients. In addition, disseminated viral infections occur in the skin lesions of AD. Though these diseases are relatively rare and little is known about their specific pathogenesis, some of them are among the true medical emergencies in dermatology. This contribution covers eczema herpeticum, the disseminated viral infection of an eczematous skin disease with the herpes simplex virus, as it is the clinically most important viral complication of AD.

History and Epidemiology

Eczema herpeticum (EH) was first described in 1887, when the Austrian dermatologist Moritz Kaposi [1] reported on 10 children with eczema larvare infantum complicated by a vesicopustular eruption. Today, the term 'Kaposi's varicelliform eruption' is used for any disseminated cutaneous infection with herpes simplex virus (HSV) type 1 or 2, which may include atopic dermatitis (AD), eczema, Darier-White disease [2], pemphigus foliaceus [3], mycosis fungoides [4], Sézary syndrome [5], ichthyosis vulgaris [6], Hailey-Hailey disease [7] and even burn patients [8]. In contrast, the term EH should be restricted to disseminated HSV infection as a complication of an eczematous skin disease [9].

The clinical presentation of EH is a disseminated, distinctly monomorphic eruption of dome-shaped vesicles, accompanied by fever, malaise and lymphadenopathy. The blisters dry out within 1–2 weeks, forming crusts that fill eroded pits. The head, neck and upper body are the most frequently affected areas. Lesions are restricted to areas of visible eczema. Mortality of disseminated HSV infection was as high as 80% prior to systemic antiviral treatment, and may be associated with viremia, multiple organ involvement and encephalitis [10, 11].

Population-based epidemiological data on EH is difficult to obtain because of its rarity. Only a few studies have investigated a larger number of patients with EH [12–14], and the predisposing factors for EH are essentially those of severe AD – an early onset of the underlying AD and a high total serum IgE level [13]. An episode of EH in an intrinsic AD patient is a clinical rarity. More than 75% of the patients with EH had not received corticosteroid treatment in the 4 weeks prior to onset of EH, arguing against a role for topical corticosteroids in the development of EH [13].

Diagnostic Procedures

Typical manifestations of EH are easily diagnosed on clinical grounds. The differential diagnosis may include widespread impetigo, eczema vaccinatum, contact dermatitis and chickenpox. The clinical diagnosis should be confirmed by polymerase chain reaction for viral DNA, by electron microscopic detection of herpes group virus from blister fluid or by commercial immunofluorescence tests for cells affected by HSV [15]. The demonstration of large multinucleated cells in the blister fluid and conventional light microscopy (Tzanck test) support the diagnosis. The optimal test depends on the clinical manifestation [13]. Differential blood count, erythrocyte sedimentation rate and body temperature may exhibit signs of viremia [13], while serum creatinine levels should be measured before starting systemic aciclovir therapy. Bacterial swabs will confirm bacterial colonization or infection with *Staphylococcus aureus* or other bacteria.

Patients with EH should be seen by an ophthalmologist to monitor for herpetic keratitis and by a neurologist if meningeal involvement or central nervous system infection is suspected because of headache or confusion [16]. A CT scan of the head, EEG and lumbar puncture should be ordered if herpes encephalitis is suspected [17].

Pathogenesis of Eczema Herpeticum

The clinical presentation of EH may be caused by primary or secondary HSV infection [13]. The higher frequency of HSV-1-induced EH, as compared to HSV-2, reflects the higher prevalence of HSV-1 in the general population.

The impaired skin barrier of AD lesions, together with the spongiosis, makes it easier for the virus to invade the skin and bind to its cellular receptors. The desmosomal protein nectin-1 has been identified as one of the relevant HSV receptors in man [18].

The increased production of Th2 cytokines in AD lesions reduce the innate immune response against HSV [19]. Abnormalities in the IFN-γ response are a risk factor for developing EH [20]. Some inducible antimicrobial peptides, and especially the antiviral cathelicidin LL-37 show defective upregulation in AD lesions [21]. This defect is relevant for EH, and cathelicidin deficiency predisposes AD patients to develop EH [22].

A patient's ability to defend himself against HSV infection may critically depend on the production of antiviral type-I IFNs. Plasmocytoid dendritic cells (PDC) are a distinctive dendritic cell subset that circulate in the blood and make up to 0.1% of peripheral blood mononuclear cells [23]. As PDC produce large amounts of antiviral type I IFN-α and IFN-β upon viral infection, their presence seems most important for the susceptibility of patients to viral skin infections [24, 25]. Compared to other inflammatory skin diseases such as psoriasis or contact dermatitis, AD patients have an impaired recruitment of PDC into their skin lesions [24]. All of these experimental data explain nicely why patients with AD show a predisposition to viral skin infections [19].

Therapy of Eczema Herpeticum

A combination of topical and systemic EH treatment is the standard of care, and should be started at the earliest time point possible. Systemic antiviral chemotherapy is the mainstay of EH treatment, and oral antibiotics are frequently added to control bacterial superinfection. Topical administration of antiseptic lotions may improve the clinical course of EH by drying out the vesicles and preventing bacterial superinfection [13].

Anti-inflammatory glucocorticosteroid therapy in acute EH stages has been a topic of controversy, as the anti-inflammatory activity is associated with an unwanted attenuation of the antiviral immune defense. Some clinicians avoid glucocorticosteroids in the acute phase of EH. In our own institution, topical and systemic steroids are freely given once systemic antiviral therapy has been started, and the results have been excellent [15].

Antiviral Chemotherapy of Eczema Herpeticum

Systemic antiviral chemotherapy is necessary to avoid the complications of disseminated HSV infection such as herpes encephalitis or herpes keratitis, and is performed with nucleoside analogues interfering with viral DNA replication. The mortality rate of EH leading to multiple organ involvement and encephalitis before the introduction of aciclovir was about 70% [10, 11].

Aciclovir is a nucleoside analogue that is metabolized in HSV-infected cells only to aciclovir-monophosphate. Further activation to aciclovir-di- and -triphosphate is catalyzed by cellular enzymes. The nucleoside triphosphate inhibits viral DNA synthesis by interaction with the DNA polymerase of HSV. Aciclovir is highly efficient and safe with systemic administration. Shortening of EH duration by oral aciclovir has been demonstrated in a multicenter, double-blind, placebo-controlled study [26]. The currently recommended regimen for EH and other severe HSV infections, such as neonatal herpes, HSV encephalitis and HSV infection in HIV patients is a 7-day course of intravenous aciclovir (3 × 5–10 mg/kg/day), which may be prolonged according to the clinical course of the disease. Oral aciclovir should be restricted to mild EH because of its lower bioavailability. Oral aciclovir prophylaxis may be considered in patients with severe recurrent EH in a dosage of 2 × 400 mg/day [16].

Aciclovir is not licensed during pregnancy, but EH during pregnancy may cause intrauterine infection of the fetus by transplacental transmission, which leads to an increased rate of abortion, death and birth defects [27]. An individual risk-benefit evaluation made for each patient will usually result in intravenous treatment with aciclovir [28]. According to the manufacturer, 1,246 pregnancy outcomes with prenatal aciclovir exposure did not show increased birth defects. Therefore, EH during pregnancy should be treated with intravenous aciclovir (3 × 5–10 mg/kg/day) for at least 7 days to avoid HSV-induced abortion, death and birth defects.

Valaciclovir is the L-valyl ester prodrug of acyclovir, and shows increased oral bioavailability as well as a more convenient dosing regimen. We recommend a 7-day course of oral valaciclovir (3 × 500 mg/day) for EH treatment, which should be prolonged according to the clinical course of the disease [29]. We recommend oral valaciclovir prophylaxis for high-risk patients at a dosage of 2 × 250 mg/day [16].

Penciclovir is a nucleoside deoxyguanosine analog that inhibits the DNA synthesis of HSV. The safety profile and antiviral activity spectrum of penciclovir is largely identical to aciclovir. Penciclovir is phosphorylated in HSV-infected cells to its triphosphate and inserted in the viral DNA in place of the nucleotide guanine, thus inhibiting virus replication. The 100-fold higher inhibitory activity of aciclovir is compensated by the longer intracellular half-life of penciclovir. Doses of 2 × 5 mg/kg/day are as effective as aciclovir in clinical trials [30].

Famciclovir, the diacetate ester derivative of 6-deoxy-penciclovir, is the oral prodrug of penciclovir and almost completely converted to penciclovir during bowl passage. Famciclovir 3 × 250 mg/day for at least 7 days has been recommend for mild clinical courses of EH [31].

Foscarnet is a phosphonate and substrate analogue of pyrophosphate formed during viral DNA synthesis. Phosphonates inhibit the viral DNA polymerase independent of thymidine kinases and are thus the treatment of choice for patients with aciclovir resistance. Intravenous foscarnet was shown to be highly effective in HIV patients with aciclovir-resistant HSV infection [32]. As it is highly nephrotoxic, foscarnet should be considered for therapy in cases of aciclovir resistance only [16].

Topical Treatment of Eczema Herpeticum

Current treatment paradigms for EH call for a combination of systemic antiviral and antibacterial substances with topical anti-inflammatory treatment. Any topical glucocorticosteroid preparation that would reasonably be applied in AD lesions of similar severity and localization is fine.

There is no evidence that the additional use of topical antiviral agents on the skin may improve the clinical course of EH in comparison to systemic antiviral chemotherapy alone. In contrast, there is evidence for contact sensitization to aciclovir, possibly resulting in drug eruptions following oral administration in sensitized individuals [33]. Due to the lack of data about treatment of EH with topical aciclovir, penciclovir or foscarnet and the potency of contact sensitization, we do not add topical antiviral agents to antiviral chemotherapy in EH except in herpetic keratitis and mucocutaneous lesions [16].

Ophthalmic Therapy

Patients with EH rarely suffer from herpetic eye disease, but those showing herpetic eyelid lesions and reduced corneal sensitivity should receive prophylactic local treatment to prevent epithelial and stromal keratitis, uveitis and secondary glaucoma [16].

Besides ophthalmic topical antiviral agents such as trifluridine, idoxuridine or brivudin, which belong to the group of 5-substituted 2′-desoxyuridines, topical formulas of the nucleoside analog aciclovir have been developed for the treatment of HSV-induced epithelial keratitis. In HSV stromal keratitis and uveitis, topical and systemic antivirals must be combined with corticosteroids to suppress the associated immune-mediated inflammation [16].

IFN Therapy for Eczema Herpeticum

Many studies on IFNs for the treatment of HSV have been performed during the last years. Two main types of IFN, type I and type II, are known: type I or 'viral' IFNs are secreted by PDC upon viral infection and include IFN-α and IFN-β, type II IFN is IFN-γ [24]. IFNs show potent antiviral properties by inhibition of virus replication and the production of virion progeny [34]. Although some studies show promising results [35–37], more studies must be performed to evaluate the efficacy and risks of IFN therapy in disseminated HSV infection and the effect of IFNs on the underlying AD.

Outlook

In spite of considerable advantages in our understanding of EH pathophysiology, the systemic use of nucleoside analogues such as acyclovir is still the mainstay of EH treatment. The introduction of this substance class has largely changed the quite unfavorable prognosis of 19th century EH to what it is today – an important and potentially lethal, but in clinical reality good manageable disease.

References

1 Kaposi M: Pathologie und Therapie der Hautkrankheiten. Vienna, Urban and Schwarzenberg, 1887.

2 Higgins CR, Schofield JK, Tatnall FM, Leigh IM: Natural history, management and complications of herpes labialis. J Med Virol 1993;suppl 1:22–26.

3 Martins-Castro R, Proenca N, de Salles-Gomes LF: On the association of some dermatoses with South American pemphigus foliaceus. Int J Dermatol 1974; 13:271–275.

4 Masessa JM, Grossman ME, Knobler EH, Bank DE: Kaposi's varicelliform eruption in cutaneous T cell lymphoma. J Am Acad Dermatol 1989;21:133–135.

5 Brion N, Guillaume JC, Dubertret L, Touraine R: Disseminated cutaneous herpes of the adult and Sezary syndrome. Ann Dermatol Venereol 1981;108: 517–521.

6 Verbov J: Fixed drug eruption due to phenazone in a hypnotic. Br J Dermatol 1972;86:438.

7 Schirren H, Schirren C, Schlupen E, Volkenandt M, Kind P: Exacerbation of Hailey-Hailey disease by infection with herpes simplex virus. Detection with polymerase chain reaction (in German). Hautarzt 1995;46:494–497.

8 Nishimura M, Maekawa M, Hino Y, Mihara K, Kohda H: Kaposi's varicelliform eruption. Development in a patient with a healing second-degree burn. Arch Dermatol 1984;120:799–800.

9 Wollenberg A, Wetzel S, Burgdorf WH, Haas J: Viral infections in atopic dermatitis: pathogenic aspects and clinical management. J Allergy Clin Immunol 2003;112:667–674.

10 Sanderson IR, Brueton LA, Savage MO, Harper JI: Eczema herpeticum: a potentially fatal disease. Br Med J (Clin Res Ed) 1987;294:693–694.

11 Wheeler CE Jr, Abele DC: Eczema herpeticum, primary and recurrent. Arch Dermatol 1966;93:162–173.

12 Bork K, Brauninger W: Increasing incidence of eczema herpeticum: analysis of seventy-five cases. J Am Acad Dermatol 1988;19:1024–1029.

13 Wollenberg A, Zoch C, Wetzel S, Plewig G, Przybilla B: Predisposing factors and clinical features of eczema herpeticum – a retrospective analysis of 100 cases. J Am Acad Dermatol 2003;49:198–205.

14 Beck LA, Boguniewicz M, Hata T, Schneider LC, Hanifin J, Gallo R, Paller AS, Lieff S, Reese J, Zaccaro D, Milgrom H, Barnes KC, Leung DY: Phenotype of atopic dermatitis subjects with a history of eczema herpeticum. J Allergy Clin Immunol 2009;124:260–9, 269.e1–7.

15 Wetzel S, Wollenberg A: Eczema herpeticatum. Hautarzt 2004;55:646–652.

16 Rerinck HC, Kamann S, Wollenberg A: Eczema herpeticatum: Pathogenese und Therapie. Hautarzt 2006;57:586–591.

17 McGrath N, Anderson N, Croxson M, Powell K: Herpes simplex encephalitis treated with acyclovir: diagnosis and long term outcome. J Neurol Neurosurg Psychiatry 1997;63:321–326.

18 Yoon M, Spear PG: Disruption of adherens junctions liberates nectin-1 to serve as receptor for herpes simplex virus and pseudorabies virus entry. J Virol 2002;76:7203–7208.

19 Wollenberg A, Klein E: Current aspects of innate and adaptive immunity in atopic dermatitis. Clin Rev Allergy Immunol 2007;33:35–44.

20 Leung DY, Gao PS, Grigoryev DN, Rafaels NM, Streib JE, Howell MD, Taylor PA, Boguniewicz M, Canniff J, Armstrong B, Zaccaro DJ, Schneider LC, Hata TR, Hanifin JM, Beck LA, Weinberg A, Barnes KC: Human atopic dermatitis complicated by eczema herpeticum is associated with abnormalities in IFN-gamma response. J Allergy Clin Immunol 2011;127:965–73 e1–5.

21 Ong PY, Ohtake T, Brandt C, Strickland I, Boguniewicz M, Ganz T, Gallo RL, Leung DY: Endogenous antimicrobial peptides and skin infections in atopic dermatitis. N Engl J Med 2002;347: 1151–1160.

22 Howell MD, Wollenberg A, Gallo RL, Flaig M, Streib JE, Wong C, Pavicic T, Boguniewicz M, Leung DY: Cathelicidin deficiency predisposes to eczema herpeticum. J Allergy Clin Immunol 2006;117:836–841.

23 Cella M, Jarrossay D, Facchetti F, Alebardi O, Nakajima H, Lanzavecchia A, Colonna M: Plasmacytoid monocytes migrate to inflamed lymph nodes and produce large amounts of type I interferon. Nat Med 1999;5:919–923.

24 Wollenberg A, Wagner M, Günther S, Towarowski A, Tuma E, Moderer M, Rothenfusser S, Wetzel S, Endres S, Hartmann G: Plasmacytoid dendritic cells: a new cutaneous dendritic cell subset with distinct role in inflammatory skin diseases. J Invest Dermatol 2002;119:1096–1102.

25 Novak N, Allam JP, Hagemann T, Jenneck C, Laffer S, Valenta R, Kochan J, Bieber T: Characterization of FcepsilonRI-bearing CD123 blood dendritic cell antigen-2 plasmacytoid dendritic cells in atopic dermatitis. J Allergy Clin Immunol 2004;114:364–370.

26 Niimura M, Nishikawa T, Martin A, Booth A, Brocklehurst P, Kinghorn G, Carney O, Helsen K, Ross E, Ellis E, Shen R, Cowan F, Mindel A: Treatment of eczema herpeticum with oral acyclovir. Am J Med 1988;85:49–52.

27 Rappersberger K: Infektionen mit Herpes-simplex und Varizella-Zoster-Viren in der Schwangerschaft. Klinische Manifestationen bei Mutter, Fötus und Neugeborenen – therapeutische Optionen. Hautarzt 1999;50:706–714.
28 Wollenberg A, Degitz K: Herpetic eczema in pregnancy (in German). Dtsch Med Wochenschr 1995; 120:1395–1398.
29 Perry CM, Faulds D: Valaciclovir. A review of its antiviral activity, pharmacokinetic properties and therapeutic efficacy in herpesvirus infections. Drugs 1996;52:754–772.
30 Lazarus HM, Belanger R, Candoni A, Aoun M, Jurewicz R, Marks L: Intravenous penciclovir for treatment of herpes simplex infections in immunocompromised patients: results of a multicenter, acyclovir-controlled trial. The Penciclovir Immunocompromised Study Group. Antimicrob Agents Chemother 1999;43:1192–1197.
31 Perry CM, Wagstaff AJ: Famciclovir. A review of its pharmacological properties and therapeutic efficacy in herpesvirus infections. Drugs 1995;50:396–415.
32 Safrin S, Crumpacker C, Chatis P, Davis R, Hafner R, Rush J, Kessler HA, Landry B, Mills J: A controlled trial comparing foscarnet with vidarabine for acyclovir-resistant mucocutaneous herpes simplex in the acquired immunodeficiency syndrome. The AIDS Clinical Trials Group. N Engl J Med 1991; 325:551–555.
33 Wollenberg A, Baldauf C, Ruëff F, Przybilla B: Allergische Kontaktdermatitis und Arzneiexanthem auf Aciclovir – Kreuzreaktion auf Ganciclovir. Allergo J 2000;9:96–99.
34 Katze M, He Y, Gale M: Viruses and interferon: a fight for supremacy. Immunology 2002;2:675–687.
35 Mikloska Z, Cunningham AL: Alpha and gamma interferons inhibit herpes simplex virus type 1 infection and spread in epidermal cells after axonal transmission. J Virol 2001;75:11821–11826.
36 Sainz B Jr, Halford WP: Alpha/Beta interferon and gamma interferon synergize to inhibit the replication of herpes simplex virus type 1. J Virol 2002;76: 11541–11550.
37 Noisakran SJ, Carr DJ: Therapeutic efficacy of DNA encoding IFN-alpha1 against corneal HSV-1 infection. Curr Eye Res 2000;20:405–412.

Prof. Dr. Andreas Wollenberg
Department of Dermatology, Ludwig Maximilian University
Frauenlobstrasse 9–11
DE–80337 Munich (Germany)
Tel. +49 89 5160 6010, E-Mail wollenberg@lrz.uni-muenchen.de

Ring J, Darsow U, Behrendt H (eds): New Trends in Allergy and Atopic Eczema.
Chem Immunol Allergy. Basel, Karger, 2012, vol 96, pp 96–99

Bone Mineral Density in Patients with Atopic Dermatitis

Inge Haeck · Sara van Velsen · Marjolein de Bruin-Weller · Carla Bruijnzeel-Koomen

Department of Dermatology/Allergology, University Medical Center Utrecht, Utrecht, The Netherlands

Abstract

In a recent investigation of bone mineral density (BMD) in patients with moderate-to-severe AD, we found that one third of the patients had a low BMD, predominately males. This could be due to the use of topical corticosteroids or due to chronic inflammation. However, neither could be held responsible for the above finding. Low BMD at baseline does not seem to progress quickly, as assessed in a 2-year follow-up study. Treatment of low BMD is questionable as the effect of vitamin D and/or calcium supplementation on low BMD is controversial. We recommend performing long-term follow-up studies to assess the course of BMD over time from onset of AD.

We recently assessed bone mineral density (BMD) in adult patients with moderate-to-severe AD [1]. We found that one third of the patients with moderate-to-severe AD were found to have low BMD. Surprisingly, it was predominately males (epidemiologically not the gender at risk) who had a low BMD [2]. BMD in AD has previously only been assessed by Aalto-Korte et al. [3]. In a study of 28 AD patients, about 11% of the patients were documented to have a Z-score less than –2. Using a cutoff value of –1 for the Z-score, the prevalence of patients with a low BMD in this study would be 42.9%, which is more in concordance with our findings.

Low BMD in AD patients may be due to absorption of topical corticosteroids or to chronic inflammation. If applied in sufficient amounts, potent topical corticosteroids can become systematically available [4–7]. This is increased when the skin barrier function is impaired, which is the case in lesional skin [8]. Therefore, chronic use of potent topical corticosteroids may lead to low BMD. However, in our cross-sectional study, there was no difference in the cumulative use of topical corticosteroids in the 5 years prior to investigation between patients with a low BMD and normal BMD, although we did find a trend towards an increased risk of low BMD with higher use of topical and oral corticosteroids. Also, in a 2-year follow-up study we found no significant difference in change of BMD between patients who had used 'low' or 'high' amounts of topical corticosteroids during a 2-year follow-up [9].

In conclusion, empirically, we found no indications that topical corticosteroid use decreases BMD. This may be explained by the relatively low amounts that have been used in our study populations. The patients described by Haeck et al. [1] used an average of 31.5 g per month and those in van Velsen et al. [9] used 86.8 g per month. In both studies, the doses were less than the safe amount advised for class III (100 g/week) or class IV (30–60 g/week) topical corticosteroids (according to Dutch guidelines) [10]. It has been shown that patients with moderate-to-severe AD on average have 9 flares of their disease per year, with each episode lasting 15 days. Zuberbier et al. [11] reported that only 54% of patients use topical corticosteroids as the main means to treat a flare, and patients endured their flare without initiating treatment for 7 days. During a disease flare, the average use of topical corticosteroids is probably more than the safe amount mentioned above, but generally it is of short duration in the majority of patients. Additionally, bone loss induced by corticosteroids is substantially reversible following withdrawal. Two prospective studies have demonstrated a reaccumulation of BMD over approximately the same time span as the loss occurred [12, 13]. This suggests that the influence of short periods during which high amounts of potent topical corticosteroids are used on BMD may be reversed during relatively long periods of low topical corticosteroid consumption, resulting in no effect on BMD overall. Furthermore, previous studies have shown that the greatest decrease in BMD is seen during the first 6 months of treatment in various diseases requiring oral corticosteroids, such as rheumatoid arthritis, sarcoidosis and systemic lupus erythematosus [14]. Bone loss continues after this period, but at a lower rate [15]. This may explain why we found only a slight decrease in BMD over time. Further follow-up studies are necessary to estimate after which time period this will become clinically relevant.

A second reason for low BMD in AD is chronic inflammation. In patients with inflammatory diseases such as rheumatoid arthritis, inflammation is an important cause of bone loss [16, 17]. Many of the cytokines (e.g. IL-1, IL-6, IL-4, IFN-γ and TNF-α) implicated in inflammatory diseases, such as in rheumatic diseases, have been demonstrated to affect osteoclast differentiation and function. This may occur either directly by acting on osteoclasts, or indirectly by acting on other cell types that influence the expression of the key osteoclastogenic factor receptor activator of NF-κB ligand (RANKL) and/or its inhibitor osteoprotegerin [17, 18]. We did not find significant differences in RANKL serum levels between patients with normal and low BMD. In our studies we did not explicitly look at disease activity/inflammation as a reason for low BMD, as it is rather difficult to assess the influence of corticosteroids and inflammation independently on BMD. This is because the use of corticosteroids will always be related to the severity of the inflammation, and there are virtually no patients with high disease activity but low use of corticosteroids. Furthermore, disease activity can fluctuate substantially in AD patients; therefore, measuring disease activity only reflects the current level of inflammation and not the inflammation over a longer period of time.

The question arises whether we should treat low BMD in AD patients. We measured vitamin D levels and found that 32% of the patients had vitamin D insufficiency (serum level <72.5 nmol/l) and 31.2% of the patients had 25-hydroxyvitamin D deficiency (serum level <50 nmol/l), which, however, was not related to low BMD. A recent review by Isenor et al. [19] did not find a clear relation between 25-hydroxyvitamin D concentration and fracture risk. Furthermore, there is inconsistency between measurement assays of 25-hydroxyvitamin D and no consensus on its optimal levels [19]. To date, the literature has shown conflicting results about the effect of calcium and vitamin D supplementation on BMD and fracture prevention [20, 21]. The inconclusiveness is also reflected by discrepancy between US and UK guidelines for patients using corticosteroids, as the US rheumatology guidelines advise supplementation of calcium plus vitamin D in all patients using corticosteroids, while the UK guidelines only advise supplementation in patients with a low dietary intake of calcium and/or vitamin D insufficiency [22]. The Dutch guidelines also advise to supplement calcium in patients with a low dietary intake during corticosteroid therapy. Therefore, measurement of vitamin D levels has little clinical usefulness at this moment and it is questionable if supplementation of calcium and/or vitamin D decreases the risk of bone loss in patients with AD.

Conclusions

BMD may be low in AD patients. We did not find a significant relation with the cumulative dose of topical corticosteroids. Since low BMD at baseline does not seem to progress quickly and the effect of vitamin D or calcium supplementation on low BMD is controversial, there are not enough reasons to screen all AD patients for low BMD. Patients with known risk factors for low BMD, such as a history of fractures and a family history of osteoporosis, are the exception. We recommend performing long-term follow-up studies to assess the course of BMD over time from onset of AD. The time course of BMD should then be compared between AD patients with severe and mild disease and healthy controls. These studies would give insight to what extent the course of BMD in (severe) AD patients is different than in people without AD, and whether screening for BMD is necessary.

References

1 Haeck I, Hamdy N, Timmer-de Mik, L, Lentjes E, Verhaar H, Knol M, de Bruin-Weller M, Bruijnzeel-Koomen C: Low bone mineral density in adult patients with moderate to severe atopic dermatitis. Br J Dermatol 2009;161:1248–1254.
2 Pietschmann P, Rauner M, Sipos W, Kerschan-Schindl K: Osteoporosis: an age-related and gender-specific disease – a mini-review. Gerontology 2009; 55:3–12.
3 Aalto-Korte K, Turpeinen M: Bone mineral density in patients with atopic dermatitis. Br J Dermatol 1997;136:172–175.
4 Munro DD: The effect of percutaneously absorbed steroids on hypothalamic-pituitary-adrenal function after intensive use in in-patients. Br J Dermatol 1976;94(suppl 12):67–76.
5 Munro DD: Topical corticosteroid therapy and its effect on the hypothalamic-pituitary-adrenal axis. Dermatologica 1976;152(suppl 1):173–180.
6 Weston WL, Fennessey PV, Morelli J, Schwab H, Mooney J, Samson C, et al: Comparison of hypothalamus-pituitary-adrenal axis suppression from superpotent topical steroids by standard endocrine function testing and gas chromatographic mass spectrometry. J Invest Dermatol 1988;90:532–535.
7 Hehir M, Du VA, Eilon L, Danie MJ, Shenoy EV: Investigation of the pharmacokinetics of clobetasol propionate and clobetasone butyrate after a single application of ointment. Clin Exp Dermatol 1983;8: 143–151.
8 Pariser D: Topical corticosteroids and topical calcineurin inhibitors in the treatment of atopic dermatitis: focus on percutaneous absorption. Am J Ther 2009;16:264–273.
9 van Velsen S, Haeck I, Knol M, Lam M, Bruijnzeel-Koomen C: Two-year follow-up of bone mineral density in adults with moderate to severe atopic dermatitis: no effect of topical cortcosteroids. J Am Acad Dermatol 2010;63:824–831.
10 Farmacotherapeutisch Kompas 2009 The Netherlands. http://www.farmacotherapeutischkompas.nl (accessed December 2009).
11 Zuberbier T, Orlow SJ, Paller AS, Taieb A, Allen R, Hernanz-Hermosa JM, et al: Patient perspectives on the management of atopic dermatitis. J Allergy Clin Immunol 2006;118:226–232.
12 Laan RF, van Riel PL, van de Putte LB, van Erning LJ, van't Hof MA, Lemmens JA: Low-dose prednisone induces rapid reversible axial bone loss in patients with rheumatoid arthritis. A randomized, controlled study. Ann Intern Med 1993;119:963–968.
13 Rizzato G, Montemurro L: Reversibility of exogenous corticosteroid-induced bone loss. Eur Respir J 1993;6:116–119.
14 LoCascio V, Ballanti P, Milani S, Bertoldo F, LoCascio C, Zanolin EM, et al: A histomorphometric long-term longitudinal study of trabecular bone loss in glucocorticoid-treated patients: prednisone versus deflazacort. Calcif Tissue Int 1998;62:199–204.
15 Saito JK, Davis JW, Wasnich RD, Ross PD: Users of low-dose glucocorticoids have increased bone loss rates: a longitudinal study. Calcif Tissue Int 1995;57: 115–119.
16 Da Silva JA, Jacobs JW, Kirwan JR, Boers M, Saag KG, Ines LB, et al: Safety of low dose glucocorticoid treatment in rheumatoid arthritis: published evidence and prospective trial data. Ann Rheum Dis 2006;65:285–293.
17 Walsh NC, Crotti TN, Goldring SR, Gravallese EM: Rheumatic diseases: the effects of inflammation on bone. Immunol Rev 2005;208:228–251.
18 Clowes JA, Riggs BL, Khosla S: The role of the immune system in the pathophysiology of osteoporosis. Immunol Rev 2005;208:207–227.
19 Isenor JE, Ensom MH: Is there a role for therapeutic drug monitoring of vitamin D level as a surrogate marker for fracture risk? Pharmacotherapy 2010;30: 254–264.
20 Buckley LM, Leib ES, Cartularo KS, Vacek PM, Cooper SM: Calcium and vitamin D3 supplementation prevents bone loss in the spine secondary to low-dose corticosteroids in patients with rheumatoid arthritis. A randomized, double-blind, placebo-controlled trial. Ann Intern Med 1996;125:961–968.
21 Adachi JD, Bensen WG, Bianchi F, Cividino A, Pillersdorf S, Sebaldt RJ, et al: Vitamin D and calcium in the prevention of corticosteroid induced osteoporosis: a 3 year follow-up. J Rheumatol 1996; 23:995–1000.
22 Compston J: Management of glucocorticoid-induced osteoporosis. Nat Rev Rheumatol 2010;6: 82–88.

Prof. Dr. Carla Bruijnzeel-Koomen
Department of Dermatology and Allergology, University Medical Centre Utrecht
G02.124, Heidelberglaan 100
NL–3584 CX Utrecht (The Netherlands)
Tel. +31 88 755 7388, E-Mail c.bruijnzeel@umcutrecht.nl

Ring J, Darsow U, Behrendt H (eds): New Trends in Allergy and Atopic Eczema.
Chem Immunol Allergy. Basel, Karger, 2012, vol 96, pp 100–107

Immunosuppressive Effect of Prolactin-Induced Protein

S. Sugiura[a] · M. Fujimiya[c] · H. Ebise[d] · Y. Miyahira[e] · I. Kato[f] · Y. Sugiura[g] · T. Kimura[d] · M. Uehara[h] · H. Sato[b] · H. Sugiura[b,i]

[a]Faculty of Medicine and [b]Department of Bioscience, Shiga University of Medical Science, Otsu, [c]Department of Anatomy, Sapporo Medical University, Sapporo, [d]Genomic Science Laboratories Dainippon Sumitomo Pharma. Co., Ltd., Osaka, [e]Division of Diagnostic Pathology, Shiga University of Medical Science Hospital, Otsu, [f]Department of Bioorganic Chemistry Faculty of Pharmaceutical Sciences Hokuriku University, Kanazawa, [g]National Center for Global Health and Medicine, Tokyo, [h]Yasu Hospital, Yasu, and [i]Sugiura Skin Clinic, Kusatsu, Japan

Abstract

Prolactin-induced protein (PIP) has been shown to bind to CD4 and is speculated to block CD4-HLA-DR interaction. However, the immunomodulatory effect of PIP on chronic allergic contact dermatitis (ACD) remains to be elucidated. The aim of this work was to define the role of PIP during the immunoresponse. Using an oxazolone-induced mouse chronic ACD model, expression of PIP was immunohistologically examined. Furthermore, effects of continued exposure of a peptide mimicking the major binding site of PIP (amino acids 106–132) for CD4 was examined in a mouse chronic ACD model. We clarified that keratinocytes and dermal infiltrating cells are positively stained with anti-PIP antibody. The PIP peptide significantly downregulated oxazolone-induced mouse ACD compared to the controls. We also found that inflammation of PIP-non-applied control ear was also suppressed in a synchronized manner in the late phase of the PIP peptide applied mouse. These findings suggest that PIP might have an immunosuppressive effect in mouse chronic ACD.

Prolactin and growth hormone causes the induction of prolactin-induced protein (PIP) in a human breast cancer cell line [1]. PIP has been detected in exocrine organs such as the bronchial epithelium and sweat, salivary and lachrymal glands; in the seminal vesicles; and corresponding fluids [2]. Human amniotic fluid also contains high concentrations of PIP. PIP was also found in breast milk [3] from normal women.

PIP specifically binds to CD4 and PIP is a specific inhibitor of T lymphocyte programmed cell death [4]. Autiero et al. [5] reported that PIP specifically binds to the CD4 domain 1. A major CD4-binding site is located between amino acids 134–148 in the β2 domain of HLA-DR, and the β2 domain of HLA-DR primarily binds to the CD4 domain 1 [6]. Autiero et al. [7] suggested that binding between PIP and CD4 blocks the CD4-HLA-DR interaction.

In allergic contact dermatitis (ACD), immunocompetent cells express HLA-DR molecules and CD4 molecules during their active phase [8, 9]. Therefore, we reasoned that PIP might modulate ACD. However, the distribution and immunological effect of PIP on ACD remain to be elucidated.

The aim of this work was to define the role of PIP during the immunoresponse. Firstly, we observed PIP expression in a low-dose oxazolone-induced mouse chronic ACD model. We also observed the effect of a synthetic peptide mouse PIP 106–132, corresponding to residues 106–132 of human PIP that constitute the major binding site for CD4, on the mouse model.

Materials and Methods

Animals

Male C57BL/6 (Japan Clea, Hamamatsu, Japan) mice between 2 and 3 months of age were used.

Induction of Oxazolone-Induced Contact Sensitivity

Mice were sensitized with a single application of 10 μl of a 1.6% solution of oxazolone (Sigma-Aldrich, St Louis, Mo., USA) on their left ear 6 days before challenge. In the experiment of repeated oxazolone challenges, each of the 6 mice were challenged with 10 μl of a 0.05% and 0.1% solution of oxazolone on the left ear.

Immunohistological Study of the Ear with Anti-Prolactin-Induced Protein Antibody in Oxazolone Challenged Mice

Twenty days after challenge, the ear samples from 12 mice were fixed with 10% neutral formaldehyde. Paraffin sections (4 μm) were incubated with a rabbit polyclonal antibody to mouse PIP/GCDFP-15 (dilution 1:1,000; Santa Cruz Biotech, Santa Cruz, Calif., USA) at 4°C overnight. Sections were then incubated with peroxidase-labeled anti-rabbit or anti-mouse antibody (Histofine Simplestain Max PO; Nichirei) for 30 min at room temperature. Peroxidase activity was detected with diaminobenzidine (Sigma-Aldrich). Sections were counterstained with hematoxylin.

Construction of Mouse Prolactin-Induced Protein Peptide

One of the strongest CD4-binding domains of human PIP was determined by Basmaciogullari et al. [7] as RTVQI AAVVDVIREL GICPDDAAVI PI. From an alignment of the mouse and human PIP gene products [10], RTVTF ATVIDIVREK NICPNDMAVV PI was identified as a CD4-binding domain of the mouse protein (59.3% homology at the amino acid level). The mouse PIP gene peptide was synthesized and used in the present mouse chronic ACD model study. As a control peptide, QD NTRKIIIKNF DIPKSVRPND EVTAVLAVQT ELK was used in the study.

Animals and Induction of Oxazolone-Induced Contact Sensitivity

Male C57BL/6 mice were challenged with 10 μl of a 0.05% solution of oxazolone on both ears four times per week (mice challenged on days 0, 2, 4, 6, 7, 9, 11, 13, 14, 16, 18, 20, 21, 23, 25) as described before.

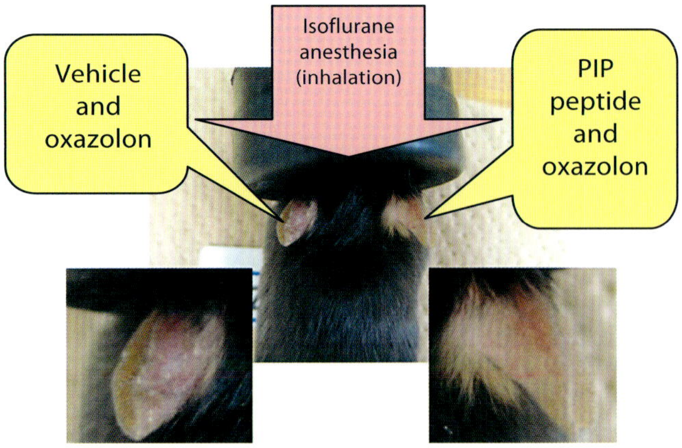

Fig. 1. Clinical feature of ear thickness at day 18. The left ear which was applied vehicle and oxazolone shows moderate erythema with scales. The right ear which was applied with PIP peptide and oxazolone shows normal color appearance and weak erythema.

Induction of an Immunomodulatory Effect by Prolactin-Induced Protein Peptide

1 μg/ml PIP Peptide Assay (6 Mice). A modulatory effect was induced by repeated topical application of the PIP peptide (10 μl of a 1 μg/ml stock solution with 0.0124% DMSO in normal saline) on the right ear. An individual mouse was treated on the left ear with 10 μl of the vehicle (0.0124% DMSO in normal saline) alone (fig. 1). Application of PIP to the right ear and vehicle to the left ear was performed a few minutes after each application of oxazolone.

25 μg/ml PIP Peptide Assay (6 Mice). Using the same protocol as described for the 1 μg/ml PIP peptide assay, 10 μl of a 25 μg/ml solution of PIP peptide with 0.31% DMSO in normal saline was applied to the right ear and 10 μl of vehicle (0.31% DMSO in normal saline) to the left ear of 6 mice.

1 and 25 μg/ml Control Peptide Assay (6 Mice Each). In the experiment involving repeated oxazolone challenges, mice were challenged with oxazolone and 10 μl of 25 μg/ml or 1 μg/ml control peptide in normal saline solution on the right ear and oxazolone and control vehicle (normal saline) on the left ear four times per week (mice challenged on days 0, 2, 4, 6, 7, 9, 11, 13, 14, 15).

Measurement of Ear Thickness and Tissue Sample Collections

Ear thickness was measured with a dial micrometer (Mitsutoyo Co., Tokyo, Japan) 24 or 48 h after each challenge. For the 1 and 25 μg/ml PIP peptide group, tissue samples from 12 mice were collected at day 18 (4 mice) after challenge during the ascending phase of ear thickness, day 21 (4 mice) at peak plateau of ear thickness and day 25 (4 mice) during the descending phase of ear thickness. The results of the time course experiment were defined by comparison with the thickness of ears receiving oxazolone alone. Tissue samples were collected 24 or 48 h after each challenge.

Histology and Immunohistochemistry of Ears on Mice Treated with Oxazolone and Prolactin-Induced Protein Peptide

Perfusion Fixation. Twelve mice were transcardially perfused with an ice-cold fixative using the same method as described [11]. Pinnae were sliced from base to apex. The slices of pinnae were processed into 4-μm paraffin sections and then stained with hematoxylin and eosin and examined by light microscopy.

Staining with Anti-Prolactin-Induced Protein Antibody. All samples obtained from the ear of each mouse were stained with anti-mouse PIP antibody as described above.

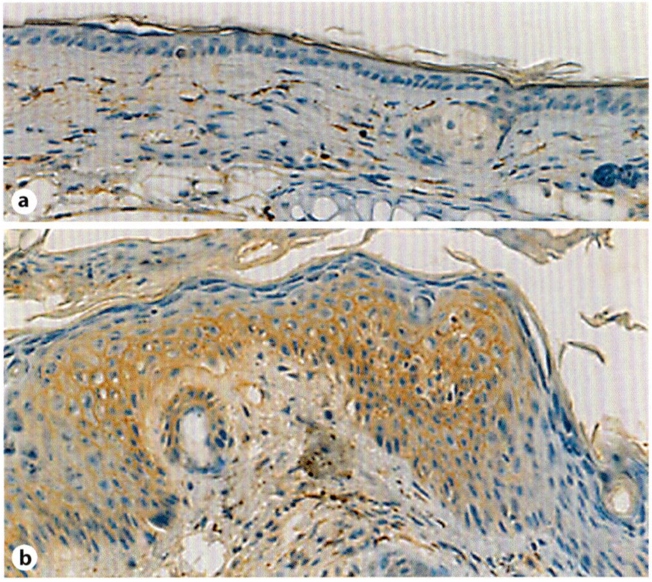

Fig. 2. Expression of PIP in skin lesions of the mouse chronic ACD model. PIP expression was absent in normal keratinocytes of the normal control mouse (**a**). In skin lesions of the ear obtained at 20 days after challenge in the oxazolone-induced chronic ACD mouse model, the cell surface of hyperplastic epidermal cells was positively stained in a reticular pattern with anti-PIP antibody (**b**).

Statistical Analyses
Differences of ear thicknesses between mice treated and untreated with PIP peptides were evaluated using a paired t test. Differences less than the false discovery rate [12] of 0.05 were considered significant.

Results

Expression of Prolactin-Induced Protein in Skin Lesions in a Mouse Chronic Allergic Contact Dermatitis Model

PIP expression was absent in normal keratinocytes of the normal control mouse (fig. 2a). In skin lesions of the ear obtained 20 days after challenge in the oxazolone-induced chronic ACD mouse model, the cell surface of hyperplastic epidermal cells was positively stained in a reticular pattern with anti-PIP antibody (fig. 2b).

Immunosuppressive Effect of Prolactin-Induced Protein Peptide in a Mouse Chronic Allergic Contact Dermatitis Model

1 µg/ml Prolactin-Induced Protein Peptide Assay (6 Mice). Figure 3a shows the mean ear thickness from day 0 to day 21. Repeated application of 1 µg/ml PIP peptide and oxazolone significantly ($p < 0.05$) inhibited the ear swelling from day 6 to day 21 compared to oxazolone alone.

25 µg/ml Prolactin-Induced Protein Peptide Assay (6 Mice). Figure 3b shows the mean ear thickness from day 0 to day 21. Repeated application of 25 µg/ml PIP peptide

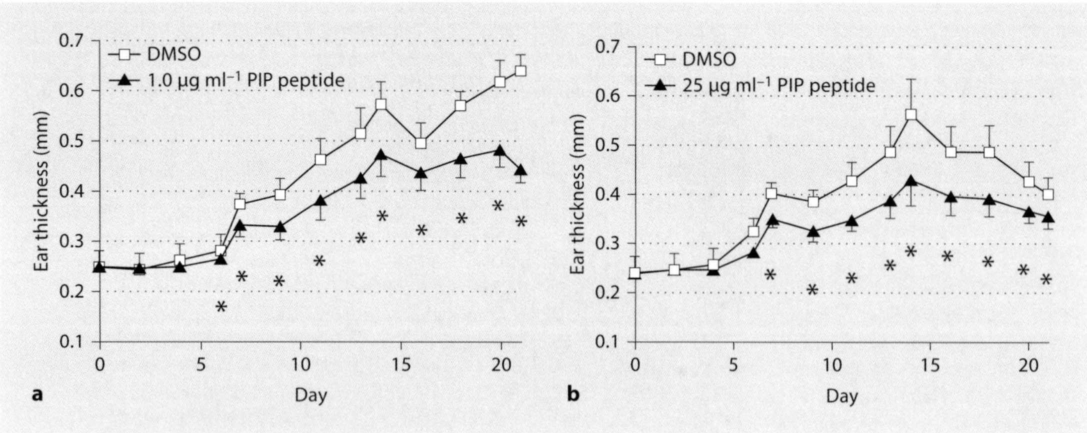

Fig. 3. Immunosuppressive effect of PIP peptide on mouse chronic ACD model. Repeated application of 1 μg/ml PIP peptide and oxazolone significantly ($p < 0.05$) inhibited the ear thickness from day 6 to day 21 compared with vehicle and oxazolone (**a**). Repeated application of 25 μg/ml PIP peptide and oxazolone significantly inhibited the ear thickness from day 7 to day 21 compared with vehicle and oxazolone. Both ears simultaneously started to decrease in thickness at day 14 (**b**).

and oxazolone significantly inhibit the ear swelling from day 7 to day 21 compared to oxazolone alone. Thus, the time course of right and left ear thickness of each mouse was strictly synchronized in mice treated with 25 μg/ml PIP peptide and oxazolone. The turning point of ear thickness on the side receiving oxazolone alone occurred earlier in mice receiving 25 μg/ml PIP peptide and oxazolone (day 14) compared with mice receiving 1 μg/ml PIP peptide and oxazolone (day 21). These findings strongly indicate that mouse PIP peptide not only has a local immunosuppressive role, but also systemically influences the level of ACD.

1 and 25 μg/ml Control Peptide Assay (6 Mice Each). A significant difference in total ear thickness was not detected between the side receiving control peptide and the untreated side in the repeated oxazolone-induced mouse ACD model.

Local Inhibitory Effect of Prolactin-Induced Protein Peptide Observed by Histopathology

Thick parakeratosis, epidermal thickening, spongiosis and infiltrates of inflammatory cells were observed in ears treated with oxazolone alone from day 18 (ascending phase; fig. 4a) to day 21 (peak plateau) after the initial challenge. A similar but much less intense reaction was seen for ears treated with oxazolone and 1 μg/ml (fig. 4b) or 25 μg/ml PIP peptide by comparison with the oxazolone alone control. At day 25 (descending phase) after challenge, both the 1 μg/ml PIP peptide group and 25 μg/ml PIP peptide group displayed very mild epidermal hyperplasia and few dermal infiltrating cells.

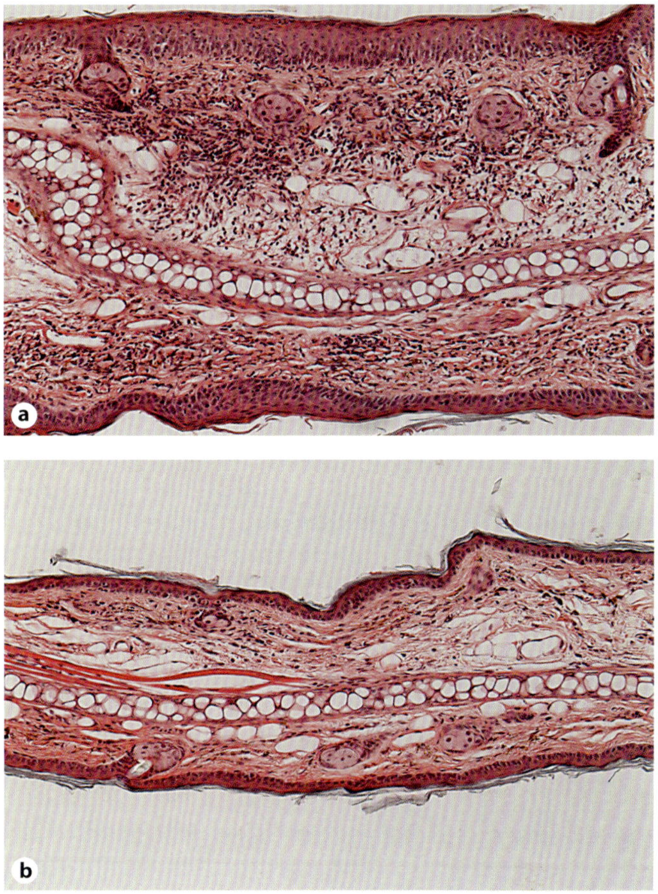

Fig. 4. Local inhibitory effect of PIP peptide observed by histopathology on day 18. The ear receiving vehicle and oxazolone shows intensive epidermal thickness and many mononuclear cells (**a**). The ear receiving 1 µg/ml PIP peptide and oxazolone shows a much less intense reaction (**b**).

Discussion

In the present study, we clarified that intrinsic PIP appears on keratinocytes in the mouse low-dose oxazolone-induced chronic ACD model. This is the first study to report that PIP is expressed on keratinocytes and infiltrating cells in the chronic phase of the immunoresponse. These findings indicate that PIP might be involved in a delayed-type hypersensitivity reaction in mouse.

The most interesting finding in our study was the definition of the immunological role of PIP. Specifically, the immunosuppression of PIP and our finding that extrinsic mouse PIP peptide intensifies the original immunosuppressive role of intrinsic PIP.

Firstly, to determine the local role of PIP in the delayed type hypersensitivity reaction, we applied a synthetic PIP peptide (amino acids 106–132) to the mouse chronic ACD model. From these experiments, we clarified that PIP peptide attenuates local chronic inflammation (fig. 3, 4). Secondly, the present study suggests that PIP and/or PIP peptide exerts a systemic immunosuppressive effect. This conclusion is supported by independent lines of evidences. First, the descending phase decrease of ear thickness observed in the ear to which PIP had not been applied was synchronized with that in the ear to which PIP had been applied (fig. 3). Second, as shown in figure 3, a high dose of PIP peptide brings about an earlier turning point of ear thickness on the side treated with oxazolone alone than a low dose of PIP peptide does. Thirdly, extrinsic PIP peptide can intensify the immunosuppressive role of intrinsic PIP. Indeed, PIP displays an immunosuppressive effect that increases in accordance with an increase of PIP peptide concentration as shown in figure 3.

As speculated by Basmaciogullari et al. [7] intrinsic PIP observed in the present study might block CD4-HLA-DR interaction.

Gaubin et al. [4] clarified that PIP is a strong and specific inhibitor of CD4/TCR-mediated apoptosis, and suggest that PIP plays a role in host defense against infections and tumors. Considering the local and systemic immunosuppressive effect of PIP observed in the present study, we additionally speculate a physiological role for the potent inhibitory effect on CD4 apoptosis, which might play a part in the long-lasting immunosuppressive effect and in preventing excessive immunoreaction.

PIP in the human amniotic fluid [2] and in the mouse oral cavity [13] is thought to provide some protective role by binding to any invading bacteria before activation of the immune system. Our results suggest that PIP, in addition to having a host defense role, also exerts a physiological protective role for excessive delayed-type hypersensitivity reaction in parts of the body where PIP is abundant, such as the oral cavity, bronchus, palms and soles.

From a clinical point of view, the itch-eliciting role of sweating in atopic dermatitis is generally accepted. Skin lesions usually deteriorate after rubbing the eyes with tears, the perioral area with saliva and the antecubital and popliteal fossae with sweat, where PIP is produced abundantly. These clinical findings are contrary to the immunosuppressive role of PIP. Currently, the reason for the discrepancy between the clinical features and immunosuppressive effect of mouse PIP is unclear.

Prolactin has been shown to stimulate many immunocompetant cells and act in maintaining immune system homeostasis [14]. Prolactin has pleiotropic actions in different organs. In the present study, we observed an immunosuppressive effect of PIP. Thus, some immune system homeostasis functions, which are known to be introduced by prolactin, might be expressed via PIP. In addition to cutaneous delayed type reaction, PIP might act as an immunomodulator in other organs such as oral cavity, bronchus, nasolaryngeal area, intestine and lachrymal related orbit area.

References

1 Murphy LC, Tsuyuki D, Myal Y, et al: Isolation and sequencing of a cDNA clone for a prolactin-inducible protein (PIP). J Biol Chem 1987;262: 15236.

2 Haagensen DE Jr, Gall SA, Brazy JE, et al: Analysis of amniotic fluid, maternal plasma, and cord blood for a human breast gross cystic disease fluid protein. Am J Obstet Gynecol 1980;138:25–32.

3 Sánchez LM, Vizoso F, Díez-Itza I, et al: Identification of the major protein components in breast secretions from women with benign and malignant breast diseases. Cancer Res 1992;52:95–100.

4 Gaubin M, Autiero M, Basmaciogullari S, et al: Potent inhibition of CD4/TCR-mediated T cell apoptosis by a CD4-binding glycoprotein secreted from breast tumor and seminal vesicle cells. J Immunol 1999;162:2631–2638.

5 Autiero M, Abrescia P, Guardiola J: Interaction of seminal plasma proteins with cell surface antigens: presence of a CD4-binding glycoprotein in human seminal plasma. Exp Cell Res 1991;197:268–271.

6 Autiero M, Houlgatte R, Martin M, et al: Competition of HLA-DR and a beta 2 domain peptide for HIV envelope glycoprotein gp120 binding to CD4. Int Immunol 1995;7:191–197.

7 Basmaciogullari S, Autiero M, Culerrier R, et al: Mapping the CD4 binding domain of gp17, a glycoprotein secreted from seminal vesicles and breast carcinomas. Biochemistry 2000;39:5332–5340.

8 Lynch GW, Slaytor EK, Elliott FD, et al: CD4 is expressed by epidermal Langerhans' cells predominantly as covalent dimers. Exp Dermatol 2003;12: 700–711.

9 Albanesi C, Cavani A, Girolomoni G: Interferon – stimulated human keratinocytes express the genes necessary for the production of peptide-loaded MHC class II molecules. J Invest Dermatol 1998;110: 138–142.

10 Myal Y, Iwasiow B, Yarmill A, et al: Tissue-specific androgen-inhibited gene expression of a submaxillary gland protein, a rodent homolog of the human prolactin-inducible protein/GCDFP-15 gene. Endocrinology 1994;135:1605–1610.

11 Nagata K, Fujimiya M, Sugiura H, Uehara M: Intracellular localization of serotonin in mast cells of the colon in normal and colitis rats. Histochem J 2001;33:559–568.

12 Benjamini Y, Hochberg Y: Controlling the false discovery rate: a practical and powerful approach to multiple testing. J R Statist Soc B 1995;57:289–300.

13 Lee B, Bowden GH, Myal Y: Identification of mouse submaxillary gland protein in mouse saliva and its binding to mouse oral bacteria. Arch Oral Biol 2002; 47:327–332.

14 Yu-Lee LY: Prolactin modulation of immune and inflammatory responses. Recent Prog Horm Res 2002;57:435–455.

Dr. Hisashi Sugiura
Department of Bioscience, Shiga University of Medical Science
Otsu 520-2192 (Japan)
Tel. +81 77 569 5702, E-Mail sugiura.clinic@iris.eonet.ne.jp, sugiurah@belle.shiga-med.ac.jp

Ring J, Darsow U, Behrendt H (eds): New Trends in Allergy and Atopic Eczema.
Chem Immunol Allergy. Basel, Karger, 2012, vol 96, pp 108–112

Is Food Allergy Testing Reliable in Pediatric Atopic Dermatitis? A Population-Based Study

Laura E. Keck · Eric L. Simpson · Trista M. Berry · Jon M. Hanifin

Department of Dermatology, Oregon Health and Science University, Portland, Oreg., USA

Abstract

We sought to assess the value and reliability of serologic testing for predicting clinical food allergy in a population-based cohort of infants with atopic dermatitis (AD). Infants 3–18 months of age, recruited from the general population, were followed quarterly for 3 years and carefully evaluated for evidence of immediate reactions to foods. Specific serum IgE levels for six foods were assayed at 3–5 years. Parents were interviewed at each visit regarding past/current immediate food-specific reactions involving skin, gut or respiratory systems. Data were entered into Excel for calculations of performance characteristics. Nine of the 40 patients (23%) who completed 3 years of follow-up had reactions to one or more foods. Reactions occurred in 5, 11 and 18% to milk, peanut and egg ingestion, respectively. In contrast, 30% of food-specific serum IgE tests were above normal. Predictive reliability of tests was generally low unless values were in the high range for peanut and milk. Conversely, egg allergy could be seen across a nearly full-spectrum of IgE values, making prediction highly unreliable. We conclude that physician and patient misinterpretation of the relevance and reliability of allergy testing may misdirect proper prevention and therapy of AD.

During the past century, the association between IgE reactivity and atopic dermatitis (AD) led to an assumption that food allergy was a causative factor. In recent years, an alternative concept has arisen, suggesting that food-specific IgE reactivity may be a secondary phenomenon caused by excessive transcutaneous absorption of antigens through a dysfunctional stratum corneum barrier [1, 2]. The concept was greatly strengthened by studies showing the strong association between filaggrin mutations, ichthyosis vulgaris, AD and asthma [3].

Well-documented food allergy prevalence among children with AD in university clinics is roughly 30%, but because of weak and inconsistent diagnostic criteria, reports may cite frequencies of 60–80% [2, 4]. Only distinct type I reactions occurring within 20–120 min of food ingestion clearly confirm the presence of food allergy. Confusing the issue are claims that a variety of delayed skin symptoms and lesions, including

Table 1. Frequency of elevated food-specific IgE levels and immediate allergic reactions among children with AD

Food	Never exposed, n (%)		Exposed, n		
	total	with increased IgE (%)	total	with increased IgE (%)	with allergy (% exposed)
Peanut	3	3 (100)	37	10 (27)	4 (10)
Egg	2	1 (50)	38	18 (47)	7 (18)
Cow milk	1	0 (0)	39	16 (41)	2 (5)
Wheat	0	0 (0)	40	13 (33)	0 (0)
Soy	4	0 (0)	36	6 (17)	0 (0)
Fish	4	0 (0)	36	4 (11)	0 (0)

eczema flares and morbilliform rashes 1–4 days later, result from food allergy. The predictive reliability of IgE testing to foods is controversial with values often reported as 'low' to 'very high' and varying with patient age and underlying health conditions [5–7]. Our objective was to evaluate the predictive reliability of food-specific IgE testing in a population-based cohort of children 3–5 years of age with AD.

Methods

Infants 3–18 months of age with mild-to-moderate AD, but no history of food or respiratory allergy, were recruited from the general population. Specific serum IgE levels for six foods (ImmunoCAP) were determined at baseline and after 3 years. Parents were interviewed quarterly regarding known exposures to each of the tested foods and for any reactions within 30–120 min of ingestion. Delayed or indeterminate reactions (e.g. eczema flares, constipation) were not accepted as indicators of allergy.

AD severity was quantitated by EASI score. IgE levels were considered elevated if >0.34 kU/l [5]. Data were entered into Excel for calculations (SPSS was used to assess correlations).

Results

A total of 88 subjects were initially screened and 40 completed 3 years, at which time 90% or more had ingested each of the six food antigens studied (table 1). Nine children had immediate type clinical reactions, consistent with true food allergy, after ingestion of one or more foods. These included reactions from exposure to egg white in 7 of 38 (18%), peanut in 4 of 37 (11%) and milk in 2 of 39 (5%). No child reacted to wheat, soy or fish, or any other foods during the 3 years of the study. Of the 240 tests performed after 3 years on study, 71 (30%) showed specific IgE above the normal level (0.34 kU/l). Even the 3 children who had never been known to ingest peanuts

Table 2. IgE decision points[1] compared to reactions in infants exposed to foods

Allergen (n)	IgE 'definitely allergic' kU/l (range)		IgE 'possibly allergic' kU/l (range)		IgE 'nonallergic' <0.35 kU/l	
	reported reaction	no reported reaction	reported reaction	no reported reaction	reported reaction	no reported reaction
Peanut (37)	4 (26.1–73)	0	0	6 (0.47–1.01)	0	27
Egg white (38)	3 (7.8–48.6)	1 (7.58)	4 (0.38–0.71)	11 (0.37–3.43)	0	19
Milk (39)	2 (>100)	0	0	14 (0.41–2.84)	0	23

[1] Decision points from Sampson [5].

had increased peanut-specific IgE ranging from 0.70 to 18.00 kU/l (mean: 7.56 kU/l), suggesting possible transcutaneous exposure [2].

We categorized specific IgE values into 'definitely allergic', 'possibly allergic' and 'nonallergic' using Sampson's risk predictions [5] (table 2). Values varied widely, leaving risk uncertain over an extensive range from low to 'definitely allergic' ranges. Patients with egg allergy were most unpredictable, ranging from 0.38 to 48.6 kU/l and levels for 4 of 7 egg-allergic patients were well below the 95% prediction level from many studies [5–8]. Values in our two milk-allergic children were very high, in the 'definitely allergic' range, while none of the 14 in the 'possibly allergic' range reacted to milk. Overall, IgE values in the 'possibly allergic' realm among our allergic patients were not indicative of allergy except for egg. Thus, 90% of values might have been wrongly assumed to be allergy. Regarding overall prevalence of elevated serum IgE in our cohort, we calculated the percentages in the normal, 'possibly reactive' and 'reactive' ranges of IgE [5]. Values indicated that only 11–50% of AD children have elevated IgE levels for the six common food allergens and, as mentioned above, even fewer showed true allergy.

Discussion

Food allergy has become a high-impact concern in many Western countries. News stories banner case reports and medical providers focus on testing and dietary avoidance strategies. Industries, including allergen producers, laboratory test manufacturers, and probiotic and hypoallergenic formula makers, all profit from the food allergy obsession. Misrepresentations are fueled by studies selected for severe AD patients in tertiary care centers and by reports implying that diagnostic criteria such as IgE tests and eczema flares are reliable indicators of food allergy. Our study profiles young children selected for treatment of AD, a group typically seen in dermatology and pediatric clinics, contrasting greatly with the many studies in selected children [5–11]. Our results suggest that diagnoses and prevalence estimates of relevant IgE sensitization and actual food allergy in infants and children with AD may be considerably inflated.

Another misapprehension from studies in AD is the belief by many that food allergy is an important causative factor for AD. Such correlative claims are not borne out by our study. Roughly 80% of our children had neither serologic nor clinical evidence of food allergy. Most patients with elevated sIgE levels had mild eczema, easily controlled with topical care. Causative misperceptions are fueled by the frequently positive skin tests and elevated serum IgE levels that may be secondary to AD barrier defects. It is reinforced by reports of eczema improvement with food restriction [11], although all agree that the natural course of AD is improvement during childhood and that restrictive diets are diagnostically unreliable [12]. Allergic causation of eczema is a strong belief among allergists, primary care physicians and alternative practitioners, which leads to extensive and often unnecessary allergy testing and, in turn, greatly amplifies the public concern about food allergy.

Our data show that the majority of positive food-specific IgE test results lie across a wide, highly uninterpretable gray zone. Too often the diagnosis of allergy is based on test values rather than history or food challenge. Our results should cause serious reconsideration about the utility of blind IgE testing among children with AD and suggests that serum IgE should not be routinely ordered in AD.

While preliminary, our report illustrates the need for a population-based prevalence study of properly defined food allergy in infants with AD [13].

Acknowledgement

The authors wish to thank Christine E. Carocci for assistance with proofreading, editing and manuscript preparation.

References

1 Simpson EL, Hanifin JM: Atopic dermatitis. Med Clin North Am 2006;90:149–167.
2 Lack G: Epidemiologic risks for food allergy. J Allergy Clin Immunol 2008;121:1331–1336.
3 Palmer CN, Irvine AD, Terron-Kwiatkowski AT, Zhao Y, Liao H, Lee SP, Goudie DR, Sandilands A, Campbell LE, Smith FJ, O'Regan GM, Watson RM, Cecil JE, Bale SJ, Compton JG, DiGiovanna JJ, Fleckman P, Lewis-Jones S, Arseculerratne G, Sergeant A, Munro CS, El Houate B, McElreavey K, Halkjaer LB, Bisgaard H, Mukhopadhyay S, McLean WH: Common loss-of-function variants of the epidermal barrier protein filaggrin are a major predisposing factor for atopic dermatitis. Nat Genet 2006;38:441–446.
4 Hill DJ, Hosking CS, de Benedictis FM, Oranje AP, Diepgen TL, Bauchau V, EPAAC Study Group: Confirmation of the association between high levels of immunoglobulin E food sensitization and eczema in infancy: an international study. Clin Exp Allergy 2007;38:161–168.
5 Sampson HA: Utility of food-specific IgE concentrations in predicting symptomatic food allergy. J Allergy Clin Immunol 2001;107:891–896.
6 Boyano Martinez T, Garcia Ara C, Diaz-Pena JM, Munoz FM, Garcia Sanchez G, Esteban MM: Validity of specific IgE antibodies in children with egg allergy. Clin Exp Allergy 2001;31:1464–1469.

7 Garcia Ara C, Boyano Martinez T, Diaz-Pena JM, Martin Munoz F, Reche Frutos M, Martin Esteban M: Specific IgE levels in the diagnosis of immediate hypersensitivity to cows' milk protein in the infant. J Allergy Clin Immunol 2001;107:185–190.
8 van der Gugten AC, den Otter M, Meijer Y, Pasmans SGAM, Knulst AC, Hoekstra MO: Usefulness of specific IgE levels in predicting cow's milk allergy. J Allergy Clin Immunol 2008;121:531–533.
9 Celik-Bilgili S, Mehl A, Verstege A, Staden U, Nocon M, Beyer K, Niggemann B: The predictive value of specific immunoglobulin E levels in serum for the outcome of oral food challenges. Clin Exp Allergy 2005;35:268–273.
10 Burks AW, Mallory SB, Williams LW, Shirrell MA: Atopic dermatitis: clinical relevance of food hypersensitivity reactions. J Pediatr 1988;113:447–451.
11 Lever R, MacDonald C, Waugh P, Aitchison T: Randomised controlled trial of advice on an egg exclusion diet in young children with atopic eczema and sensitivity to eggs. Pediatr Allergy Immunol 1998;9:13–190.
12 Chafen JJ, newberry SJ, Riedl MA, Bravata DM, Maglione M, Suttorp MJ, et al: Diagnosing and managing common food allergies: a systematic review. JAMA 2010;203;1848–1856.
13 NIAID-Sponsored Expert Panel, Boyce JA, Assa'ad A, Burks AW, Jones SM, Sampson HA, Wood RA, Plaut M, Cooper SF, Fenton MJ, Arshad SH, Bahna SL, Beck LA, Byrd-Bredbenner C, Camargo CA Jr, Eichenfield L, Furuta GT, Hanifin JM, Jones C, Kraft M, Levy BD, Lieberman P, Luccioli S, McCall KM, Schneider LC, Simon RA, Simons FE, Teach SJ, Yawn BP, Schwaninger JM: Guidelines for the diagnosis and management of food allergy in the United States: report of the NIAID-sponsored expert panel. J Allergy Clin Immunol 2010;126(6 suppl):S1–S58.

Dr. Jon M. Hanifin
Department of Dermatology (CH16D), Oregon Health and Science University
3303 S.W. Bond Avenue
Portland, OR 97239-4501 (USA)
Tel. +1 503 494 2121, E-Mail hanifinj@ohsu.edu

Ring J, Darsow U, Behrendt H (eds): New Trends in Allergy and Atopic Eczema.
Chem Immunol Allergy. Basel, Karger, 2012, vol 96, pp 113–119

New Strategies for Dealing with *Staphylococcus aureus* Colonization and the Emerging Methicillin-Resistant *Staphylococcus aureus* Epidemic in Atopic Dermatitis

Mark Boguniewicz

Division of Pediatric Allergy-Immunology, Department of Pediatrics, National Jewish Health and University of Colorado School of Medicine, Denver, Colo., USA

Abstract

Atopic dermatitis is a common inflammatory skin disease and a global health problem. Patients are often colonized or infected by *Staphylococcus aureus*, usually by toxin-producing strains. Methicillin-resistant *S. aureus* (MRSA) has emerged as an important pathogen. Community-acquired MRSA, a frequent cause of skin and soft tissue infections has become epidemic. Basic skin care measures emphasizing repair and protection of the skin barrier reduce microbial colonization and decrease the need for specific antimicrobial therapy even in patients colonized by MRSA. Novel approaches directed at *S. aureus* colonization and prevention of infection include compounds mimicking antimicrobial peptides, vaccines targeting unique antigens and toxin-neutralizing agents.

Atopic dermatitis (AD) is an inflammatory skin disorder with high prevalence rates in both developed and developing countries [1]. Patients with AD have a unique predisposition for being heavily colonized or infected by *Staphylococcus aureus* [2]. The Hanifin and Rajka criteria for AD published in 1980 recognized the tendency of AD patients to develop cutaneous infections [3]. In recent years, methicillin-resistant *S. aureus* (MRSA) has emerged as an increasingly important pathogen worldwide [4].

Community-Acquired Methicillin-Resistant *Staphylococcus aureus*

Community-acquired (CA)-MRSA was initially reported in healthy children in the late 1990s. Since then, CA-MRSA has become epidemic with skin and soft tissue

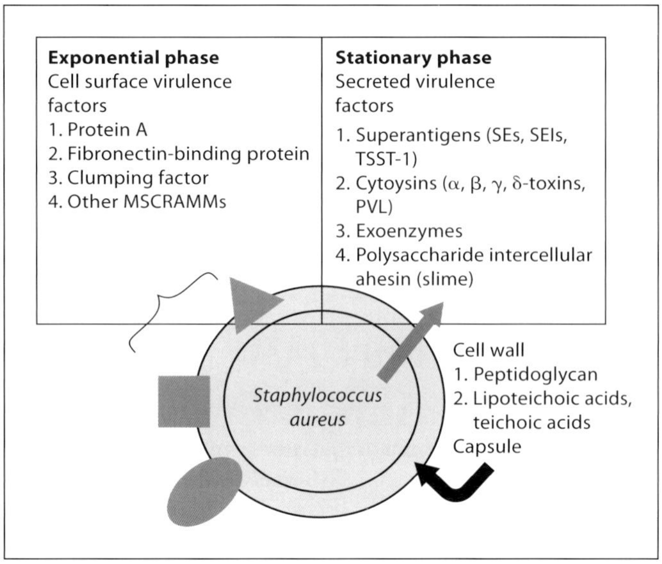

Fig. 1. Virulence factor production by *S. aureus* (reproduced with permission from Schlievert et al. [13]).

infections making up the most frequent forms of the disease [5]. In the United States, a single clone of CA-MRSA (USA 300 ST8) has become the most prevalent cause of staphylococcal skin and soft tissue infections acquired in the community, causing not only skin and soft tissue infections, but also invasive diseases [6]. Strains have been remarkable for combining antibiotic resistance with exceptional virulence and transmissibility [7]. CA-MRSA has replaced hospital-acquired MRSA as causes of serious fatal infections such as necrotizing fasciitis or Waterhouse-Friderichsen syndrome [8]. Of interest, CA-MRSA evolved from highly pathogenic methicillin-sensitive *S. aureus* strains by acquisition of methicillin resistance elements likely acquired from *Staphylococcus epidermidis*, which suggests an important role for this commensal organism as a reservoir for horizontal transmission of genetic factors [9].

Why Is Community-Acquired Methicillin-Resistant *Staphylococcus aureus* So Virulent?

Panton-Valentine leukocidin was initially thought to be the major determinant of virulence of CA-MRSA [10]. However, more recent studies have failed to support this finding [11]. Novel cytolytic peptides, alpha-type phenol-soluble modulins, appear to be important in virulence [12]. In addition, the most common CA-MRSA (USA 300) has a mobile genetic element termed ACME (arginine catabolic mobile element) that contributes to enhanced colonization by affecting pH homeostasis. Besides producing the highly inflammatory cytolysins, MRSA isolates also produce enterotoxins with superantigenic properties including enterotoxin-like Q and a highly pyrogenic deletion variant of toxic shock syndrome toxin-1 (reviewed in depth in [13]) (fig. 1). Cell-surface virulence factors also include microbial surface components recognizing adhesive matrix molecules (MSCRAMMs), which function as receptors in human hosts.

Staphylococcus aureus, Toxins and Atopic Dermatitis

Cho et al. [14] found high levels of *S. aureus* even on normal-appearing skin of AD patients not seen in psoriatic and healthy skin, and showed binding via MSCRAMMs to fibrinogen and fibronectin that appear to be preferentially expressed in AD stratum corneum. As reviewed by Schlievert et al. [13], most AD patients are colonized by toxin-secreting strains of *S. aureus*. At present, approximately 25% of isolates from moderate-severe AD patients admitted to the AD program at National Jewish Health in Denver, Colorado, are MRSA (author's unpubl. observations). Of note, both MRSA and methicillin-sensitive *S. aureus* secrete alpha-toxin critical for survival on skin. A unique finding in *S. aureus* isolates from AD patients is that approximately 10% produce two or more superantigenic toxins, whereas coproduction was not observed in isolates from more than 5,000 patients with toxic shock syndrome [13]. Of clinical importance, use of topical corticosteroids [15] and topical calcineurin inhibitors [16] both reduce staphylococcal colonization in AD patients. However, given their history of remarkable adaptability and rapid development of resistance, one concern with regular use of topical anti-inflammatory medications in AD would be selecting for strains of *S. aureus* that adapt to their new skin surface niche by increasing their virulence capabilities. Susceptibility to staphylococcal colonization and infections, including with MRSA will be a key focus of the recently NIH-funded Atopic Dermatitis Research Network.

Strategies for Dealing with Methicillin-Resistant *Staphylococcus aureus* Colonization in the Community Setting

Approaches to minimizing the impact of MRSA in the community was the subject of a comprehensive review of therapeutic strategies by a panel of experts convened by the Centers for Disease Control and Prevention [17]. Decolonization regimens employed in MRSA outbreaks in community settings have included combinations of topical and systemic antimicrobial agents and antiseptic body washes, making it difficult to evaluate the effectiveness of any individual component. Data suggest that intranasal mupirocin can be effective at eliminating *S. aureus* colonization in the short term; however, recolonization is common. Effectiveness of decolonization therapy of any kind for preventing *S. aureus* infections in individual patients has not been well established. Few data are available on the effectiveness of decolonization regimens to eliminate colonization or prevent infection in community settings or within families. Complicating matters further, adherence with decolonization regimens has been suboptimal in community settings. Development of resistance to systemic and topical agents during decolonization therapy has been reported, causing concern about widespread use of these interventions.

In patients with AD, recolonization after a course of systemic antimicrobial therapy occurs rapidly, often with the same toxin-producing strains [18]. Interventions to reduce *S. aureus* in the management of AD were the subject of a Cochrane review [19]. No benefit was found for antibacterial soaps, antibacterial bath additives or topical antibiotics/antiseptics. Adding antibiotics to topical steroids (betamethasone plus neomycin vs. clobetasol, prednicarbate and antimicrobial vs. prednicarbate, or betamethasone valerate and gentamicin vs. betamethasone) reduced numbers of *S. aureus* in several trials, but no evidence of clinical benefit was seen in other trials. One trial with 30 patients showed no significant improvement in eczema with the use of silver textiles despite using 10 times the amount of topical steroids. The authors of the Cochrane review failed to find clear evidence of benefit for antimicrobial interventions for patients with AD, despite their widespread use [19]. This does not necessarily mean they do not work because the studies were small and not optimally designed, pointing to the need for larger studies with long-term outcomes. In addition, use of antiseptics in managing patients with AD was recently reviewed [20]. Of note, a controlled study of dilute bleach baths with intermittent intranasal mupirocin showed decreased clinical severity of AD in patients with clinical signs of secondary bacterial infection although the number of MRSA-positive patients was small (see review by Paller [this vol., pp. 132–140]) [21]. In the AD program at National Jewish Health in Denver, Colorado, the primary focus is on skin barrier repair utilizing an intense supervised regimen of hydration, topical anti-inflammatory medications and wet wrap therapy for the most severe patients, including those who are heavily colonized with MRSA [22].

Novel Approaches to Dealing with Resistant *Staphylococcus aureus*

Ceragenins are synthetic cationic steroid molecules that mimic endogenous antimicrobial peptides and can disrupt bacterial membranes without damaging mammalian cell membranes [23, 24]. They possess broad-spectrum activities against multidrug-resistant bacteria. Due to their synthetic nature, ceragenins are not subject to human protease degradation and therefore have a longer tissue half-life. Two of these compounds, CSA-8 and CSA-13, have been shown to be active against clinical isolates of vancomycin-intermediate *S. aureus,* heterogeneous vancomycin-intermediate *S. aureus* and vancomycin-resistant *S. aureus* compared to antibiotics such as daptomycin, linezolid and vancomycin by susceptibility testing and killing curve analysis [25].

Prior clinical trials with monovalent vaccines against *S. aureus* were not successful and newer strategies have included polyvalent formulas and targeted clinically relevant antigens [26]. Combinatory vaccines targeting MSCRAMMs demonstrated complete protection from lethal doses of *S. aureus* in a murine challenge model and were shown to prevent colonization [27]. In a different approach, researchers from Cologne, Germany, used an intravenous immunoglobulin preparation as a source of antibodies directed against anchorless *S. aureus* surface proteins for identification of vaccine candidates [28]. Subtractive proteome analysis of *S. aureus* anchorless cell wall proteins was performed and three of these candidate proteins [enolase (Eno), oxoacyl reductase (Oxo) and hp2160] were expressed as glutathione S-transferase fusion proteins. Use of affinity-purified anti-Eno, anti-Oxo and anti-hp2160 antibodies resulted in opsonization, phagocytosis and killing of *S. aureus* by human neutrophils. In addition, high specific antibody titers were detected in mice immunized with recombinant antigens. In mice challenged with bioluminescent *S. aureus*, reduced staphylococcal spread was measured by in vivo imaging. The recovery of *S. aureus* colony-forming units from organs of immunized mice was diminished 10- to 100-fold and mice immunized with hp2160 displayed statistically significant higher survival rates after lethal challenge with clinically relevant *S. aureus* strains. This data suggests that anchorless cell wall proteins might be efficacious vaccine candidates.

Given the pathogenicity of *S. aureus* toxins, a unique strategy involves engineering binding affinity agents capable of neutralizing these superantigens. Soluble forms of the engineered Vβ proteins produced in *Escherichia coli* were shown to be effective inhibitors of SEB-mediated T cell activation, and completely neutralized the lethal activity of SEB in animal models [29]. Further, this group was able to express Vβ domains in tandem as a single-chain protein and neutralized SEB and TSST-1 with a single agent, demonstrating the feasibility of neutralizing multiple toxins [30].

Conclusions

Patients with AD have skin barrier and immune abnormalities and a unique propensity to be colonized or infected by microbes, especially toxin-secreting *S. aureus*, including MRSA. Management of AD should include basic skin care with emphasis on repair and protection of the skin barrier with proper hydration and topical therapy, which includes both moisturizers and anti-inflammatory medications. Of note, these measures reduce microbial colonization and decrease the need for specific antimicrobial therapy even in patients colonized by MRSA. In patients suspected of having an infectious complication of AD, obtaining culture and sensitivities from patients with difficult-to-treat AD can help identify resistant organisms and direct antimicrobial therapy if needed. Novel approaches dealing with *S. aureus* colonization and prevention of infection include compounds mimicking antimicrobial peptides, vaccines targeting unique antigens and toxin-neutralizing agents.

References

1 Odhiambo JA, Williams HC, Clayton TO, Robertson CF, Asher MI, ISAAC Phase Three Study Group: Global variations in prevalence of eczema symptoms in children from ISAAC Phase Three. J Allergy Clin Immunol 2009;124:1251-8.e23.

2 Boguniewicz M, Leung DY: Recent insights into atopic dermatitis and implications for management of infectious complications. J Allergy Clin Immunol 2010;125:4–13.

3 Hanifin JM, Rajka G: Diagnostic features of atopic dermatitis. Acta Derm Venereol Suppl (Stockh) 1980;92:44–47.

4 Boucher HW, Corey GR: Epidemiology of methicillin-resistant *Staphylococcus aureus*. Clin Infect Dis 2008;46:S344–S349.

5 Klevens RM, Morrison MA, Nadle J, Petit S, Gershman K, Ray S, Harrison LH, Lynfield R, Dumyati G, Townes JM, Craig AS, Zell ER, Fosheim GE, McDougal LK, Carey RB, Fridkin SK, Active Bacterial Core Surveillance (ABCs) MRSA Investigators: Invasive methicillin-resistant *Staphylococcus aureus* infections in the United States. JAMA 2007;298:1763–1771.

6 Stryjewski ME, Chambers HF: Skin and soft tissue infections caused by community acquired methicillin resistant *Staphylococcus aureus*. Clin Infect Dis 2008;46:S368–S377.

7 Chambers HF: Community-associated MRSA – resistance and virulence converge. N Engl J Med 2005;352:1485–1487.

8 Miller LG, Perdreau-Remington F, Rieg G, Mehdi S, Perlroth J, Bayer AS, Tang AW, Phung TO, Spellberg B: Necrotizing fasciitis caused by community-associated methicillin-resistant *Staphylococcus aureus* in Los Angeles. N Engl J Med 2005;352:1445–1453.

9 Otto M: Community-associated MRSA: a dangerous epidemic. Future Microbiol 2007;2:457–459.

10 Vandenesch F, Naimi T, Enright MC, Lina G, Nimmo GR, Heffernan H, Liassine N, Bes M, Greenland T, Reverdy ME, Etienne J: Community-acquired methicillin-resistant *Staphylococcus aureus* carrying Panton-Valentine leukocidin genes: worldwide emergence. Emerg Infect Dis 2003;9:978–984.

11 Voyich JM, et al: Is Panton-Valentine leukocidin the major virulence determinant in community-associated methicillin-resistant *Staphylococcus aureus* disease? J Infect Dis 2006;194:1761–1770.

12 Wang R, Braughton KR, Kretschmer D, et al: Identification of novel cytolytic peptides as key virulence determinants for community-associated MRSA. Nat Med 2007;13:1510–1514.

13 Schlievert PM, Strandberg KL, Lin YC, Peterson ML, Leung DY: Secreted virulence factor comparison between methicillin-resistant and methicillin-sensitive *Staphylococcus aureus*, and its relevance to atopic dermatitis. J Allergy Clin Immunol 2010;125: 39–49.

14 Cho SH, Strickland I, Boguniewicz M, Leung DY: Fibronectin and fibrinogen contribute to the enhanced binding of *Staphylococcus aureus* to atopic skin. J Allergy Clin Immunol 2001;108:269–274.

15 Stalder JF, Fleury M, Sourisse M, Rostin M, Pheline F, Litoux P: Local steroid therapy and bacterial skin flora in atopic dermatitis. Br J Dermatol 1994;131: 536–540.

16 Remitz A, Kyllönen H, Granlund H, Reitamo S: Tacrolimus ointment reduces staphylococcal colonization of atopic dermatitis lesions. J Allergy Clin Immunol 2001;107:196–197.

17 Gorwitz RJ, Jernigan DB, Powers JH, Jernigan JA, and Participants in the CDC-Convened Experts' Meeting on Management of MRSA in the Community. Strategies for clinical management of MRSA in the community: Summary of an experts' meeting convened by the Centers for Disease Control and Prevention. 2006. Available at http://www.cdc.gov/ncidod/dhqp/ar_mrsa_ca.html. Accessed December 12, 2011.

18 Boguniewicz M, Sampson H, Leung SB, Harbeck R, Leung DY: Effects of cefuroxime axetil on *Staphylococcus aureus* colonization and superantigen production in atopic dermatitis. J Allergy Clin Immunol 2001;108:651–652.

19 Birnie AJ, Bath-Hextall FJ, Ravenscroft JC, Williams HC: Interventions to reduce *Staphylococcus aureus* in the management of atopic eczema. Cochrane Database Syst Rev 2008;3:CD003871.

20 Wollenberg A, Schnopp C: Evolution of conventional therapy in atopic dermatitis. Immunol Allergy Clin N Am 2010;3:351–368.

21 Huang JT, Abrams M, Tlougan B, Rademaker A, Paller AS: Treatment of *Staphylococcus aureus* colonization in atopic dermatitis decreases disease severity. Pediatrics 2009;123:e808–e814.

22 Boguniewicz M, Nicol NH, Kelsay K, Leung DYM: A multidisciplinary approach to evaluation and treatment of atopic dermatitis. Semin Cut Med Surg 2008;27:115–127.

23 Savage PB, Li C, Taotafa U, Ding B, Guan Q: Antibacterial properties of cationic steroid antibiotics. FEMS Microbiol Lett 2002;217:1–7.

24 Ding B, Taotofa U, Orsak T, Chadwell M, Savage PB: Synthesis and characterization of peptide-cationic steroid antibiotic conjugates. Org Lett 2004;6:3433–3436.

25 Chin JN, et al: Antimicrobial activities of ceragenins against clinical isolates of resistant *Staphylococcus aureus*. Antimicrob Agents Chemother 2007;51: 1268–1273.

26 Otto M: Targeted immunotherapy for staphylococcal infections: focus on anti-MSCRAMM antibodies. BioDrugs 2008;22:27–36.

27 Stranger-Jones YK, Bae T, Schneewind O: Vaccine assembly from surface proteins of *Staphylococcus aureus*. Proc Natl Acad Sci USA 2006;103:16942–16947.

28 Glowalla E, Tosetti B, Kronke M, Krut O: Proteomics-based identification of anchorless cell wall proteins as vaccine candidates against *Staphylococcus aureus*. Infect Immun 2009;77:2719–2729.

29 Buonpane RA, Churchill HRO, Moza B, Sundberg EJ, Peterson ML, Schlievert PM, et al: Neutralization of staphylococcal enterotoxin B by soluble, high-affinity receptor antagonists. Nat Med 2007;13: 725–729.

30 Yang X, Buonpane RA, Moza B, Nur-ur Rahman AKM, Wang N, Schlievert PM, et al: Neutralization of multiple staphylococcal superantigens by a single-chain protein consisting of affinity-matured, variable domain repeats. J Invest Dermatol 2008;198: 344–348.

Dr. Mark Boguniewicz
National Jewish Health
1400 Jackson Street, Room J310
Denver, CO 80206 (USA)
Tel. +1 303 398 1617, E-Mail boguniewiczm@njhealth.org

Ring J, Darsow U, Behrendt H (eds): New Trends in Allergy and Atopic Eczema.
Chem Immunol Allergy. Basel, Karger, 2012, vol 96, pp 120–125

Anti-IL-4 as a New Strategy in Allergy

Carsten B. Schmidt-Weber

Zentrum Allergie und Umwelt (ZAUM), Technische Universität und Helmholtz Zentrum München, Munich, Germany

Abstract

Allergic diseases are characterized by an overreaction characterized by Th2-type cell response, and as a consequence, an IgE-switched B cell immunity. Obviously, type-2 cytokines (IL-4, IL-5, IL-9, IL-13) and particularly IL-4 have been identified as potential targets for allergy treatment. While initial experiences using anti-IL-4 principles in asthma were rather ambiguous, more recent studies using an IL-4 mutein blocking the IL-4 and IL-13 receptor have shown promising results. Furthermore, our understanding of IL-4 biology is more specific and may promote more targeted interventions. A key function of IL-4 is the induction of 'master switch' transcription factor GATA3 that drives Th2 differentiation and also effectively inhibits the induction of regulatory T cells. Consequences for treatment of allergic diseases are also discussed.

The demand for novel, long-lasting and cost-effective drugs is increasing as the prevalence rate of allergies rises. IL-4 is probably one of the oldest obvious drug targets of the immune system, as it precedes the switch of immature IgM^+ to mature IgE^+ B cells. However, the switch also requires cell contact to T cells via CD40 interactions, which emphasizes the important role of allergen-specific T cells. These typically IL-4-producing Th2 cells require IL-4 themselves to differentiate from allergen-unexperienced naive T cells. The Th2-driving IL-4 may be derived from basophils [1–3], eosinophils, natural killer cells or mast cells [4–6] upon IgE-mediated cross-linking of individuals already sensitized. The classical 'chicken or the egg' causality problem concerns where in nonsensitized individuals IL-4 comes from in the first place? Recent studies indicate that novel type-2 innate immune cells ('nuocytes') are able to produce IL-4 in response to IL-25 and IL-33 [7, 8]. Although these cells remain to be detected in man, it is likely that these cells provide a key bystander role in initial allergic sensitization and are thus a target of anti-IL-4 strategies.

IL-4 Receptors and Cellular Targets

The role of IL-4 is, however, not restricted to differentiation of T and B cells. IL-4 is also recognized by nonimmune cells such as endothelial cells, cells of the placenta and multiple epithelial cells [9–16]. The IL-4 receptor complexes are heterodimers that are formed by IL-4Rα and the common γγchain (IL-2Rγ; type I IL-4R) or the IL-13Rα1 chain (type II IL-4R). IL-4Rα chains are ubiquitously expressed. IL-13 is recognized by a heterodimer of the IL-4Rα and IL-13Rα1 (type II IL-4R). IL-13Rα1 is expressed on hematopoietic cells, such as B cells, monocytes and basophils, as well as epithelial cells, endothelial cells, fibroblasts and smooth muscle cells. The shared use of IL-4Rα along with the more limited distribution of IL-13Rα1 expression, explains much of the pattern of shared and divergent biological activities of IL-4 and IL-13. Because of receptor chain sharing, it is difficult to separate whether IL-4 or IL-13 is the more relevant ligand of these structural cells. Of note, IL-13 antibodies are currently being tested in clinical trials targeting allergic diseases [17].

New Concepts and Targets

Known targeted functions of IL-4 are the above-mentioned IgE production and Th2 differentiating ability. In addition, it has an antiapoptotic role and promotes FceR1 expression, differentiation processes in monocytic/dendritic cells, mucin and eotaxin production in epithelial cells, and myofibroblast phenotypes (for review see [17]).

A nonpathogenic role of IL-4 is the control of parasitic infections, where Th2 cells play an effector role that promotes type-2 mediated inflammation [18]. Some parasites such as helminths prevent the induction of an effective Th2 immunity by promoting the induction of regulatory T cells and, thus, tolerance induction against parasitic antigens by a yet unknown mechanism [19]. This example highlights that the effective polarization of Th2 cells is critically important for tolerance regulation. We [20] and others [21–23] have demonstrated that a key function of IL-4 is the inhibition of FOXP3 and, thus, de novo induction of regulatory T cells. The mechanism underlying this inhibition is the GATA3-mediated inhibition of the *Foxp3* promoter [20]. In addition, the IL4-induced PU.1 transcription factor contributes towards the inhibition of *Foxp3* gene expression [23]. Of note, the IL-4-induced GATA3 is not the only transcription factor that inhibits FOXP3; we could observe similar mechanisms for the Th17-factor RORC2, which also inhibits FOXP3 induction [24]. In more general terms, these experiments suggest that 'inflammation prevents tolerance induction', which represents a clinical observation that is older than the discovery of regulatory T cells (fig. 1).

Allergic inflammation provides IL-4 by multiple cell types in the presence of specific allergen-recognition by Th2 cells, IgE-triggered basophils, eosinophils and mast cells, and the absence of allergens (nuocytes, natural killer cells, trophoblasts). Therefore, allergic conditions could promote loss of tolerance by providing IL-4 in a

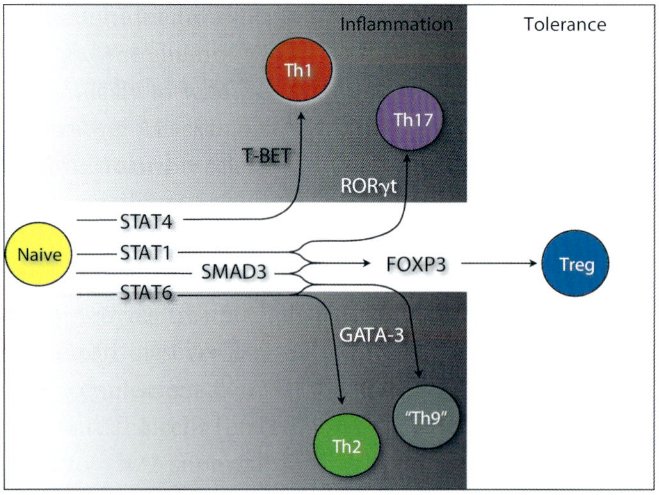

Fig. 1. Inflammation prevents allergen tolerance. The scheme illustrates the concept that regulatory T cells may evolve as default pathways upon antigen activation, as they may occur permanently when we are exposed to autoantigens or components of foreign, but harmless, commensals or allergens. Only the activation of 'danger' signals may induce transcription factors that skew the polarization process towards effector T cell phenotypes. It is noteworthy that most of the transcription factors are coexpressed in early differentiation and only disappear in later phases of T cell differentiation. STAT4 is posttranslationally activated after IL-12 engagement, while STAT6 is mobilized by IL-4 and STAT1 by IL-6 and TNF; SMAD3 responds to TGF-β. The more downstream factors are also transcriptionally regulated and can be more abundant in committing or terminally differentiated cells. Novel subsets such as Th22 are not depicted as their differentiation pathway is still unknown.

'bystander' manner. It is thus interesting to speculate that IL-4 is the mediator of the allergic march, characterized by increasing intolerance to different allergen sources and involvement of different organs.

Potential Side Effects

A cause of concern in any clinical trial is the secretion of IL-4 by trophoblasts in the placenta, which is assumed to be involved in tolerance regulation during pregnancy [25–27]. Therefore, neutralization of IL-4 may in some way interfere with pregnancy. Furthermore, the induction of IgG4 is also IL-4-dependent and may dysregulate early tolerance induction since IgG4 is assumed to compete with IgE.

Target of Anti-IL-4 Therapy

To date, clinical trials targeting IL-4 have shown moderate success. Pascolizumab is an anti-IL-4 mAb that was used for asthma; however, despite successful phase I studies

[28, 29], it was not further developed. A soluble IL-4R (blocking IL-4 and IL-13) was tested in a phase II study in patients suffering from moderate-to-severe asthma, which showed improvement only in some parameters such as decreased number of and time to exacerbations [30], but not in FEV_1. Promising results were obtained using an IL-4 mutein (pitrakinra), which represents an IL-4 protein that carries several mutations that increase the affinity to IL-4R and blocks further binding of IL-4 and IL-13. Both subcutaneous and inhalative administration significantly improved airway function (FEV_1) after 4 weeks of treatment with twice daily inhalations or once daily injections [31]. Interestingly, atopic eczema also appears to improve upon pitrakinra treatment [32]. The mechanistic background of the IL-4 mutein is unclear and it is not clear whether the beneficial effects are based on IL-13-mediated effects or on disruption of IL-4-mediated differentiation of T and B cells. Since the differentiation of these cells also requires the activation by the allergen, we hypothesize that IL-4 neutralization may be most effective in the frame of specific immunotherapy, where the allergen-driven induction of regulatory T cells is assumed to be a key step in the generation of allergen-specific immunotolerance. A clinical trial was initiated to investigate the intradermal late-phase response to allergen upon combination treatment of grass extracts with an anti-IL4 drug (VAK694; NIH clinical trials.gov: NCT01018693). An ambitious panel of secondary endpoints will inform us whether it is possible to reprogram specific immunity by combining allergen vaccination and biologicals.

Conclusion

Recent anti-IL4 therapies have shown promising success in treatment of allergic diseases. The improved understanding of IL-4 biology and functions will specify when, where and in which patients anti-IL-4 will be most effective. Successful reprogramming of type-2 immunity remains a key hurdle that will be an attractive accomplishment for the sustained and cost-effective treatment of allergic disease.

References

1 van Panhuys N, Prout M, Forbes E, Min B, Paul WE, Le Gros G: Basophils are the major producers of IL-4 during primary helminth infection. J Immunol 2011;186:2719–2728.

2 Denzel A, Maus UA, Rodriguez Gomez M, Moll C, Niedermeier M, Winter C, Maus R, Hollingshead S, Briles DE, Kunz-Schughart LA, Talke Y, Mack M: Basophils enhance immunological memory responses. Nat Immunol 2008;9:733–742.

3 Brunner T, Heusser CH, Dahinden CA: Human peripheral blood basophils primed by interleukin 3 (IL-3) produce IL-4 in response to immunoglobulin E receptor stimulation. J Exp Med 1993;177:605–611.

4 Sherman MA: The role of STAT6 in mast cell IL-4 production. Immunol Rev 2001;179:48–56.

5 Barata LT, Ying S, Meng Q, Barkans J, Rajakulasingam K, Durham SR, Kay AB: IL-4- and IL-5-positive T lymphocytes, eosinophils, and mast cells in allergen-induced late-phase cutaneous reactions in atopic subjects. J Allergy Clin Immunol 1998;101:222–230.
6 Brown MA, Pierce JH, Watson CJ, Falco J, Ihle JN, Paul WE: B cell stimulatory factor-1/interleukin-4 mRNA is expressed by normal and transformed mast cells. Cell 1987;50:809–818.
7 Barlow JL, McKenzie AN: Nuocytes: expanding the innate cell repertoire in type-2 immunity. J Leukoc Biol 2011;90:867–874.
8 Neill DR, Wong SH, Bellosi A, Flynn RJ, Daly M, Langford TK, Bucks C, Kane CM, Fallon PG, Pannell R, Jolin HE, McKenzie AN: Nuocytes represent a new innate effector leukocyte that mediates type-2 immunity. Nature 2010;464:1367–1370.
9 Ueta M, Sotozono C, Kinoshita S: Expression of interleukin-4 receptor alpha in human corneal epithelial cells. Jpn J Ophthalmol 2011;55:405–410.
10 White SR, Martin LD, Stern R, Laxman B, Marroquin BA: Expression of IL-4/IL-13 receptors in differentiating human airway epithelial cells. Am J Physiol Lung Cell Mol Physiol 2010;299: L681–L693.
11 Van Den Berg JG, Aten J, Chand MA, Claessen N, Dijkink L, Wijdenes J, Lakkis FG, Weening JJ: Interleukin-4 and interleukin-13 act on glomerular visceral epithelial cells. J Am Soc Nephrol 2000;11: 413–422.
12 van der Velden VH, Naber BA, Wierenga-Wolf AF, Debets R, Savelkoul HF, Overbeek SE, Hoogsteden HC, Versnel MA: Interleukin 4 receptors on human bronchial epithelial cells. An in vivo and in vitro analysis of expression and function. Cytokine 1998; 10:803–813.
13 Henriques CU, Rice GE, Wong MH, Bendtzen K: Immunolocalisation of interleukin-4 and interleukin-4 receptor in placenta and fetal membranes in association with pre-term labour and pre-eclampsia. Gynecol Obstet Invest 1998;46:172–177.
14 Brinckmann R, Topp MS, Zalan I, Heydeck D, Ludwig P, Kuhn H, Berdel WE, Habenicht JR: Regulation of 15-lipoxygenase expression in lung epithelial cells by interleukin-4. Biochem J 1996;318: 305–312.
15 Prens E, Hegmans J, Lien RC, Debets R, Troost R, van Joost T, Benner R: Increased expression of interleukin-4 receptors on psoriatic epidermal cells. Am J Pathol 1996;148:1493–1502.
16 Thornhill MH, Kyan-Aung U, Haskard DO: IL-4 increases human endothelial cell adhesiveness for T cells but not for neutrophils. J Immunol 1990;144: 3060–3065.
17 Steinke JW: Current prospective of anti-IL-4, -IL-9, and -IL-13 therapies in allergic disease. Recent Pat Inflamm Allergy Drug Discov 2010;4:222–230.
18 Patel N, Kreider T, Urban JF Jr, Gause WC: Characterisation of effector mechanisms at the host:parasite interface during the immune response to tissue-dwelling intestinal nematode parasites. Int J Parasitol 2009;39:13–21.
19 Wilson MS, Taylor MD, Balic A, Finney CA, Lamb JR, Maizels RM: Suppression of allergic airway inflammation by helminth-induced regulatory T cells. J Exp Med 2005;202:1199–1212.
20 Mantel PY, Kuipers H, Boyman O, Rhyner C, Ouaked N, Ruckert B, Karagiannidis C, Lambrecht BN, Hendriks RW, Crameri R, Akdis CA, Blaser K, Schmidt-Weber CB: GATA3-driven Th2 responses inhibit TGF-beta1-induced FOXP3 expression and the formation of regulatory T cells. PLoS Biol 2007;5:e329.
21 Hill JA, Hall JA, Sun CM, Cai Q, Ghyselinck N, Chambon P, Belkaid Y, Mathis D, Benoist C: Retinoic acid enhances Foxp3 induction indirectly by relieving inhibition from CD4+CD44hi cells. Immunity 2008;29:758–770.
22 Bruno L, Mazzarella L, Hoogenkamp M, Hertweck A, Cobb BS, Sauer S, Hadjur S, Leleu M, Naoe Y, Telfer JC, Bonifer C, Taniuchi I, Fisher AG, Merkenschlager M: Runx proteins regulate Foxp3 expression. J Exp Med 2009;206:2329–2337.
23 Prochazkova J, Fric J, Pokorna K, Neuwirth A, Krulova M, Zajicova A, Holan V: Distinct regulatory roles of transforming growth factor-beta and interleukin-4 in the development and maintenance of natural and induced CD4+ CD25+ Foxp3+ regulatory T cells. Immunology 2009;128:e670–e678.
24 Burgler S, Mantel PY, Bassin C, Ouaked N, Akdis CA, Schmidt-Weber CB: RORC2 is involved in T cell polarization through interaction with the FOXP3 promoter. J Immunol 2010;184:6161–6169.
25 Torricelli M, Voltolini C, Bloise E, Biliotti G, Giovannelli A, De Bonis M, Imperatore A, Petraglia F: Urocortin increases IL-4 and IL-10 secretion and reverses LPS-induced TNF-alpha release from human trophoblast primary cells. Am J Reprod Immunol 2009;62:224–231.
26 Chaouat G, Cayol V, Mairovitz V, Dubanchet S: Localization of the Th2 cytokines IL-3, IL-4, IL-10 at the fetomaternal interface during human and murine pregnancy and lack of requirement for Fas/Fas ligand interaction for a successful allogeneic pregnancy. Am J Reprod Immunol 1999;42:1–13.
27 Hill JA, Polgar K, Anderson DJ: T-helper 1-type immunity to trophoblast in women with recurrent spontaneous abortion. JAMA 1995;273:1933–1936.

28 Hart TK, Blackburn MN, Brigham-Burke M, Dede K, Al-Mahdi N, Zia-Amirhosseini P, Cook RM: Preclinical efficacy and safety of pascolizumab (SB 240683): a humanized anti-interleukin-4 antibody with therapeutic potential in asthma. Clin Exp Immunol 2002;130:93–100.
29 Shames RS, Vexler V, Lane NM, McClellan M, Shi J, Keller S, Young DY, Nieman RB, Hart T: The safety and pharmacokinetics of SB240683 (anti-IL-4 humanized monoclonal antibody) in patients with mild to moderate asthma. J Allergy Clin Immunol 2001;107:1.
30 Corren J, Busse W, Meltzer EO, Mansfield L, Bensch G, Fahrenholz J, Wenzel SE, Chon Y, Dunn M, Weng HH, Lin SL: A randomized, controlled, phase 2 study of AMG 317, an IL-4Ralpha antagonist, in patients with asthma. Am J Respir Crit Care Med 2010;181:788–796.
31 Wenzel S, Wilbraham D, Fuller R, Getz EB, Longphre M: Effect of an interleukin-4 variant on late phase asthmatic response to allergen challenge in asthmatic patients: results of two phase 2a studies. Lancet 2007;370:1422–1431.
32 Antoniu SA: Pitrakinra, a dual IL-4/IL-13 antagonist for the potential treatment of asthma and eczema. Curr Opin Investig Drugs 2010;11:1286–1294.

Prof. Dr. Carsten B. Schmidt-Weber
Zentrum Allergie und Umwelt (ZAUM), Technische Universität und Helmholtz Zentrum München
Biedersteiner Strasse 29
DE–80802 Munich (Germany)
Tel. +49 89 4140 3450, E-Mail csweber@tum.de

Ring J, Darsow U, Behrendt H (eds): New Trends in Allergy and Atopic Eczema.
Chem Immunol Allergy. Basel, Karger, 2012, vol 96, pp 126–131

New Drug Targets in Atopic Dermatitis

Dagmar Simon[a] · Hans-Uwe Simon[b]

[a]Department of Dermatology, Inselspital, Bern University Hospital, and [b]Institute of Pharmacology, University of Bern, Bern, Switzerland

Abstract

Atopic dermatitis (AD) is a chronic inflammatory skin disorder characterized by eczematous skin lesions, pruritus and typical histopathological features. T cells are thought to play a key role, but B cells might also participate in the pathogenesis of AD. In two investigator-initiated pilot studies, we studied the effects of B cell depletion by monoclonal anti-CD20 antibody therapy or a reduction of activated T cells by LFA3-IgG fusion protein on moderate-to-severe AD. All patients treated with either rituximab or alefacept showed an improvement of their skin symptoms with a sustained effect after treatment. In both studies, histological alterations, such as spongiosis, acanthosis and dermal infiltrate, including T and B cell numbers, dramatically improved and the expression of IL-5 and IL-13 was reduced after therapy. Upon rituximab therapy, allergen-specific IgE levels were not altered and total serum IgE levels only slightly decreased. According to recent studies, neutralizing B and T cells products such as IgE or IL-5 might be effective in subgroups of patients with AD.

Biologics targeting B and T cells appear to be promising in patients with severe AD. Moreover, treatment with these biologics has provided new insights into the pathogenesis of atopic dermatitis (AD).

AD is a chronic inflammatory skin disorder based on a genetic predisposition towards an impaired skin barrier and a Th2-biased immune reaction [1]. So far, the treatment of AD has consisted of immunosuppressive substances, e.g. corticosteroids, calcineurin inhibitors and cyclosporine, in combination with emollients in order to reduce inflammation and restore the defective barrier. Biological agents (biologics) present a relatively new group of therapeutics created by biological processes that include recombinant therapeutic proteins such as antibodies or fusion proteins. Biologics specifically target inflammatory cells and mediators. In AD, biologics are used in order to reduce inflammation by modulating the number, activation and function of immune cells or the action of cytokines or disease relevant antibodies (fig. 1). A number of pilot studies and retrospective analyses on the effect of biologics

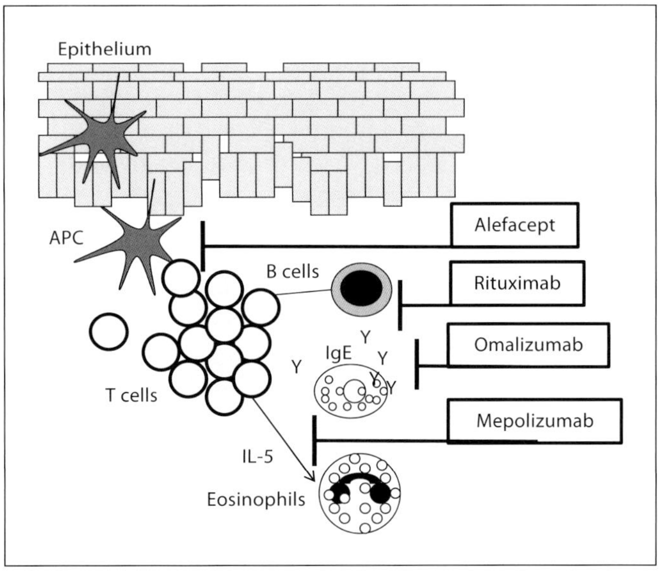

Fig. 1. B cells, T cells and their products as targets for biologics in AD.

in patients with moderate-to-severe AD refractory to topical and/or systemic therapy have been published recently. However, representative, randomized, placebo-controlled studies evaluating the efficacy and safety of biologics in AD are still not available.

Targeting B Cells

In AD, the inflammatory infiltrate consists predominantly of T cells, but variable numbers of B cells, mast cells and eosinophils are also present [2]. In 80% of AD patients, elevated levels of total IgE levels and/or specific IgE to environmental allergens are found [1]. Furthermore, Langerhans cells of AD skin bear the high-affinity IgE receptor on their surface, providing a strong link between environmental allergen exposure and T cell activation [1].

Rituximab is a chimeric monoclonal anti-CD20 antibody that eliminates B cells [3]. CD20 is expressed by pre-B cells and mature B cells, but not plasma cells. Recent studies have reported the efficacy of rituximab in the treatment of autoimmune diseases [4].

We conducted an investigator-initiated, open-label, pilot study investigating the effects of rituximab in patients with moderate-to-severe AD not responding to topical corticosteroid and/or calcineurin inhibitor therapy [5]. Rituximab (MabThera; Roche Pharma AG, Switzerland) was administered twice, each 1,000 mg i.v., 2 weeks apart.

All 6 patients (4 female, age: 19–63 years) had a significant improvement of their AD lesions within 4 weeks of treatment and further improved with a sustained effect at week 24. The pruritus scores decreased in parallel with the EASI scores. All patients reduced the application of topical corticosteroids.

The immunophenotyping of lymphocytes revealed that the number of CD20+ cells dropped down to zero within 3 days, and started to return at week 24. Interestingly, specific IgE to environmental allergens were not altered and total IgE levels were only slightly reduced after therapy (2,145 ± 662 vs. 1861 ± 612 kU/l, $p = 0.067$).

In skin biopsies taken after treatment, the histology showed an impressive improvement of hyperkeratosis, acanthosis, spongiosis and dermal infiltration, comparable with findings usually seen in nonlesional skin of AD. Upon therapy with rituximab, a marked decrease of T and B cells, but not of eosinophils and mast cells, was observed. In parallel, the numbers of cytokine-expressing CD4+ and CD8+ T cells were reduced after therapy. In agreement with these data, we observed a relative decrease in IL-5 (mean 53%) and IL-13 (mean 83%) mRNA expression. Only marginal changes were seen in IFN-γ and IL-10 mRNA expression (both were reduced by 16%) [5].

Targeting T Cells

Alefacept is a fusion protein composed of the first extracellular domain of LFA-3 (CD58) and human Ig G1 fragment crystallizable (Fc) domain [6]. Binding of the LFA-3 domain to CD2 blocks costimulation and, subsequently, activation of T cells. Furthermore, by binding to CD2 and Fcγ receptor III (CD16), alefacept mediates cognate interaction between T cells and natural killer cells resulting in T cell apoptosis.

We initiated an open-label, pilot study investigating the effects of alefacept in patients with moderate-to-severe AD not responding to adequate topical therapy [7]. Patients received 12 weekly intramuscular injections of 15 mg alefacept (Amevive®; Biogen-Dompé, Switzerland).

All 10 patients (6 females, age: 19–51 years) experienced a significant improvement upon alefacept therapy. The EASI levels continuously decreased over the treatment period and remained low or decreased further during the follow-up period until week 22. In parallel, the pruritus significantly decreased. All patients could drastically reduce the application of topical corticosteroids. Three patients were able to stop the usage of any concomitant AD medication.

Upon alefacept therapy, the numbers of T cells as well as B cells and eosinophils in the skin were significantly reduced. Measuring mRNA expression of cytokines in atopic eczema skin revealed a decrease of 75% for IL-5, 50% for IL-13, and 25% for IFN-γ and IL-10. This decrease was due to a decrease of CD4+ and CD8+ T cells expressing the cytokines IL-5, IL-10, IL-13 or IFN-γ [7].

Targeting B and T Cell Products

The inflammation in AD is characterized by a Th2 cytokine expression including IL-5 and eosinophil infiltration. The effect of a short-term therapy with the anti-IL-5 antibody mepolizumab was tested in a randomized, placebo controlled study [8]. Two injections of mepolizumab, each 750 mg, were given 2 weeks apart. After 4 weeks, a moderate improvement of clinical symptoms was observed. Interestingly, a rapid depletion of eosinophils in the peripheral blood was noted [8]. Mepolizumab had no effect on atopy patch test reactions [9]. Based on the promising results in AD and the experiences in bronchial asthma therapy, long-term trials with anti-IL-5 antibodies seem indicated.

The majority of AD patients have elevated serum IgE levels, but the pathogenic role of IgE in AD remains unknown. The first case reports gave inconsistent results on the effect of anti-IgE antibody (omalizumab) treatment in severe AD [10, 11]. Upon low-dose anti-IgE therapy with 10 cycles of 150 mg omalizumab, 6 of 11 AD patients with serum IgE levels >1,000 kU/l before therapy responded as shown by a decrease of SCORAD more than 50% in 2 patients and between 25 and 50% in 4 patients [12]. Several studies reported that accompanying AD significantly improved in patients receiving omalizumab because of severe bronchial asthma [13–15]. A recent published placebo-controlled, double-blind pilot study revealed no effect of omalizumab therapy over 16 weeks on the clinical course in AD patients. Anti-IgE therapy was demonstrated to decrease free and cell-bound IgE in the peripheral blood, reduce FcεRI expression on peripheral blood mononuclear cells, and lower the number of IgE-positive cells in the skin. Omalizumab-treated patients showed less response upon allergen challenge skin tests [16].

Discussion

These studies demonstrate that biologics are effective in the treatment of moderate-to-severe AD. Therapy with both alefacept and rituximab resulted in an improvement of symptoms and reduction of pruritus during the treatment period and had a sustained effect [5, 7]. The therapy with both biologics was well tolerated and no severe adverse events were observed.

In agreement with the dual function of alefacept, we observed decreased numbers of skin T cells and reduced T cell activation upon therapy. Alefacept therapy had anti-inflammatory effects by reducing the number of CD4+ and CD8+ T cells as well as IL-5 and IL-13 cytokine expression in the skin. The results underline the dominant role of T cells as effector immune cells in AD.

Furthermore, B cells were identified as key players in the pathogenesis of AD. The efficacy of rituximab could not simply be explained by a reduction of IgE titers. Instead, our data imply that the loss of the antigen-presenting and immunomodulatory functions of B cells might be responsible for the beneficial clinical effects.

Targeting IgE seemed to be effective in subgroups of patients with AD, such as children and those with accompanying asthma [10–15]. The observed slight-to-moderate effects of anti-IL-5 therapy in AD might be due to redundant effects of other cytokines and/or short period of therapy [8].

Biologics targeting B cells and T cells appear to be promising in patients with severe AD. Moreover, treatment with these biologics has provided new insights into the pathogenesis of AD.

Acknowledgements

We are indebted to S. Hösli, J. Wittwer, G. Kostylina, E. Kozlowski and E. Seger, who provided excellent technical support. This work was supported by research grants from Biogen-Dompé AG (Zug, Switzerland) and Roche Pharma AG (Reinach, Switzerland).

References

1 Bieber T: Atopic dermatitis. N Engl J Med 2008;358:1483–1494.
2 Simon D, Vassina E, Yousefi S, Kozlowski E, Braathen L, Simon HU: Reduced dermal infiltration of cytokine-expressing cells in atopic dermatitis following short-term topical tacrolimus treatment. J Allergy Clin Immunol 2004;114:887–895.
3 Grillo-Lopez AJ, White CA, Varns C, Shen D, Wei A, McClure A, Dallaire BK: Overview of the clinical development of rituximab: first monoclonal antibody for the treatment of lymphoma. Semin Oncol 1999;26:66–73.
4 De Vita S, Zaja F, Sacco S, De Candia A, Fanin R, Ferraccioli G: Efficacy of selective B cell blockade in the treatment of rheumatoid arthritis: evidence for a pathogenic role of B cells. Arthritis Rheum 2002;46:2029–2033.
5 Simon D, Hösli S, Kostylina G, Yawalkar N, Simon HU: Anti-CD20 (rituximab) treatment improves atopic eczema. J Allergy Clin Immunol 2008;121:122–128.
6 Miller GT, Hochman PS, Meier W, Tozard R, Bixler S, Rosa M, Wallner BP: Specific interaction of lymphocyte function-associated antigen 3 with CD2 can inhibit T cell responses. J Exp Med 1993;178:211–222.
7 Simon D, Wittwer J, Kostylina G, Büttiker U, Simon HU, Yawalkar N: Alefacept (LFA-3/IgG fusion protein) treatment for atopic eczema. J Allergy Clin Immunol 2008;122:423–424.
8 Oldhoff JM, Darsow U, Werfel T, Katzer K, Wulf A, Laifaoui J, Hijnen DJ, Plötz S, Knol EF, Kapp A, Bruijnzeel-Koomen CA, Ring J, de Bruin-Weller MS: Anti-IL-5 recombinant humanized monoclonal antibody (mepolizumab) for the treatment of atopic dermatitis. Allergy 2005;60:693–696.
9 Oldhoff JM, Darsow U, Werfel T, Bihari IC, Katzer K, Laifaoui J, Plötz S, Kapp A, Knol EF, Bruijnzeel-Koomen CA, Ring J, de Bruin-Weller MS: No effect of anti-interleukin-5 therapy (mepolizumab) on the atopy patch test in atopic dermatitis patients. Int Arch Allergy Immunol 2006;141:290–294.
10 Lane JE, Cheyney JM, Lane TN, Kent DE, Cohen DJ: Treatment of recalcitrant atopic dermatitis with omalizumab. J Am Acad Dermatol 2006;54:68–72.
11 Krathen RA, Hsu S: Failure of omalizumab for treatment of severe adult atopic dermatitis. J Am Acad Dermatol 2005;53:338–340.
12 Belloni B, Ziai M, Lim A, Lemercier B, Sbornik M, Weidinger S, Andres C, Schnopp C, Ring J, Hein R, Ollert M, Mempel M: Low-dose anti-IgE therapy in patients with atopic eczema with high serum IgE levels. J Allergy Clin Immunol 2007;120:1223–1225.
13 Sheinkopf LE, Rafi AW, Do LT, Katz RM, Klaustermeyer WB: Efficacy of omalizumab in the treatment of atopic dermatitis: a pilot study. Allergy Asthma Proc 2008;29:530–537.

14 Vigo PG, Girgis KR, Pfuetze BL, Critchlow ME, Fisher J, Hussain I: Efficacy of anti-IgE therapy in patients with atopic dermatitis. J Am Acad Dermatol 2006;55:168–170.
15 Incorvaia C, Pravettoni C, Mauro M, Yacoub MR, Tarantini F, Riario-Sforza GG: Effectiveness of omalizumab in a patient with severe asthma and atopic dermatitis. Monaldi Arch Chest Dis 2008;69:78–80.
16 Heil PM, Maurer D, Klein B, Hultsch T, Stingl G: Omalizumab therapy in atopic dermatitis: depletion of IgE does not improve the clinical course – a randomized, placebo-controlled and double blind pilot study. J Dtsch Dermatol Ges 2010;8:990–998.

Dr. Dagmar Simon
Department of Dermatology, Inselspital, Bern University Hospital
CH–3010 Bern (Switzerland)
Tel. +41 31 632 2278, E-Mail dagmar.simon@insel.ch

Ring J, Darsow U, Behrendt H (eds): New Trends in Allergy and Atopic Eczema.
Chem Immunol Allergy. Basel, Karger, 2012, vol 96, pp 132–140

Latest Approaches to Treating Atopic Dermatitis

Amy S. Paller

Departments of Dermatology and Pediatrics, Northwestern University Feinberg School of Medicine, Chicago, Ill., USA

Abstract

Recent investigations have shown atopic dermatitis (AD) results from the interplay of epidermal barrier defects, immune dysfunction and environmental triggers. These discoveries teach the importance of addressing all of these factors in treating patients. The barrier issues remind us of the need for moisturizers, especially after bathing, to replenish lipids and decrease water loss. Addition of dilute sodium hypochlorite (bleach) to bathwater often improves the dermatitis of children with moderate-to-severe dermatitis, especially with a history of staphylococcal infection. Oral vitamin D_3 has been suggested to increase the deficient antimicrobial peptide that results from cutaneous inflammation, although studies to date are inconclusive. Topical corticosteroids and calcineurin inhibitors continue to predominate as therapy and, to date, their safety record seems good, despite the Black Box warning issued in the United States. Poor compliance may explain the failure to respond to therapy, and contact dermatitis from topical application of emollients and medications may mimic AD, erroneously suggesting recalcitrance. For patients with severe AD, administration of systemic immunosuppressants may be required; ongoing studies of newer agents, including biologics, may revolutionize therapy for individuals with severe dermatitis, providing more targeted therapy in the future.

Atopic dermatitis (AD), one of the most common skin disorders seen in infants and children, now has a prevalence of almost 20% in the United States, Europe and Japan, in contrast to a prevalence of up to 3% in 1960. The increasing prevalence of AD parallels the increase noted in children with asthma, suggesting shared triggers and is consistent with the frequent development of other atopic disorders in children with AD. In fact, the initial occurrence of AD before asthma and allergic rhinitis has led to the description of an 'atopic march' to asthma and allergic rhinitis [1]. During the past 20 years, most investigations of the pathomechanism of AD have focused on cutaneous immune dysregulation as a primary defect ('inside-outside' view), and the disorder has been classified into IgE-associated (extrinsic) and non-IgE-associated (intrinsic) forms. Given that 80% of patients ultimately develop increased IgE levels and the more recent demonstration that IgE-mediated sensitization develops after the onset of disease blurs the etiologic distinction between the 'extrinsic' and 'intrinsic' forms, and suggests other important pathomechanisms [2]. During the last 5 years, new data have linked AD with defects in the epidermal barrier, leading to a new view of AD as a disorder of barrier dysfunction ('outside-inside' view) [3]. Regardless of one's stance on the relative importance of barrier or immune activation in the skin, recent discoveries teach us of the importance of addressing *both* the barrier defect and immune activation in our approach to patients, and these discoveries have translated into new ideas for bathing and moisturizing, use of antimicrobial agents, and topical anti-inflammatory therapy.

Impairment of the Epidermal Barrier: Proteins, Proteases and Lipids

Dry skin, a hallmark of AD, is related to increased transepidermal water loss, reflecting barrier dysfunction. This barrier dysfunction is also thought to allow the penetration of high-molecular-weight allergens, such as dust mite antigens, foods and microbes. The molecular basis for the barrier defect is a vigorous area of investigation, and genetic and acquired deficits in the expression of key epidermal proteins and lipids have been demonstrated.

A decrease in the epidermal granular layer and its predominant protein, filaggrin, has long been recognized as a feature of ichthyosis vulgaris, the most common disorder of cornification. The discovery in 2006 of loss-of-function mutations in profilaggrin *(FLG)* allowed the subsequent investigations proving that the clinical observation of a strong association between AD and ichthyosis vulgaris had a molecular basis. Distinct mutations in *FLG* have been discovered in European and Japanese populations, but all are strongly linked with AD, particularly of early onset [4]. Indeed, *FLG* mutations are identified in up to 30% of European patients with AD, in contrast to approximately 10% of the Northern European population overall. The linkage of AD and asthma, but not asthma alone [5], with mutations of *FLG* supports the concept of the 'atopic march' in which AD is the initial atopic disease during infancy with the later occurrence of other atopic conditions dependent on early allergen exposure through the abnormal epidermis.

Although genetic deficiency of filaggrin clearly contributes to a significant subset of individuals with AD, immunologic abnormalities further contribute to barrier abnormalities. The expression of Th2 cytokines IL-4 and IL-13 is known to suppress filaggrin expression, perpetuating a cyclic process of barrier disruption in individuals with AD [6]. In addition, genetic defects in barrier proteins in AD likely extend beyond those in filaggrin. Recently, knockout mice without loricrin, another barrier protein, were shown to have more allergen-specific antibodies, cutaneous dendritic cells and skin thickening than littermates after topical antigen exposure. In addition, the stratum corneum in lesional versus nonlesional skin shows decreased expression of other proteins related to skin barrier (corneodesmosin, desmoglein 1, desmocollin and TGM-3) [7].

The epidermal barrier can also be compromised by increased activation of epidermal proteases. Netherton syndrome, a rare disorder with AD-like features, is the prototype of poor epidermal barrier function that results from activation of serine proteases. In fact, increased serine protease (kallikrein) expression and activation have been demonstrated in the stratum corneum and serum of patients with AD [8]. Kallikrein 5, which is activated at higher skin pH, has now been demonstrated to trigger an inflammatory cascade in which proteinase-activated receptor 2 and thymic stromal lymphopoietin (TSLP) are intermediates [9]. TSLP is produced by keratinocytes and found in both acute and chronic lesions. Its expression is increased by injury and exposure to bacteria or inflammatory cytokines [9]. TSLP has been shown to instruct dendritic cells to induce a Th2 response and subsequently Th0/Th1 responses, as are seen in AD, suggesting a key role for TSLP in AD [10]. Indeed, anti-TSLP antibody blocks skin inflammation after an ovalbumin challenge and circulating TSLP is increased in children with AD, regardless of disease severity and IgE levels. Recent studies in mouse models have provided evidence that the skin delivers signals for allergic sensitization in the gastrointestinal tract and lungs, which suggests that systemic delivery of TSLP from keratinocytes is key to the development of asthma [11].

The lipid lamellae of the epidermis are formed by the secretion of lamellar granules from granular cells into the extracellular matrix. Four major lipid groups are found in the stratum corneum: ceramides, cholesterol, fatty acids and cholesterol esters. Individuals with AD show a decrease in total ceramides [12]. Liquid chromatography with electrospray ionization-mass spectrometry has now demonstrated 350 species among 11 groups of human ceramides, revealing the complexity of the lipid barrier of epidermis and promising to provide more specific definition of lipid abnormalities in the near future. Early studies suggest that specific ceramides are deficient in AD, while others are actually increased as a function of barrier impairment [13, 14].

Translation of Discoveries about Barrier Dysfunction into New Therapy

Clinicians have long understood the importance of bathing and vigorous use of emollients in AD. These new data suggest that the irritation of soaps may, in part, result from their raising of skin pH and activation of proteases, further contributing to barrier dysfunction and activating the inflammatory cascade that includes proteinase-activated receptor 2 and TSLP. pH may be particularly important in the face of filaggrin deficiency. In fact, the pH at the skin surface is higher in mice with AD related to Flg mutations (pH 5.8) versus mice with AD without Flg mutations (5.6) and in wild-type littermate skin (5.5) [14]. At least in part, this higher pH may relate to a deficit in breakdown products of filaggrin, particularly urocanic acid and pyrrolidone carboxylic acid, which are humectants and lower skin pH. The recently demonstrated decrease in expression of enzymes involved in generation of these 'natural moisturizing factors' (caspase 14, arginase, γ-glutamyl cyclotransferase) may further contribute to the deficit [7]. While these natural moisturizing factors may well become commercially available in the future, skin acidification with lactobionic acid has been shown to improve AD in a mouse model. In these studies, the decrease in skin surface pH was associated with decreases in cellular infiltration and IgE levels, as well as increases in lipid secretion and antimicrobial activity [15]. Interestingly, urocanic acid and pyrrolidone carboxylic acid have been shown to decrease the growth of *S. aureus* [15], suggesting a further link between bacterial colonization and infection and barrier dysfunction (see below).

While adjusting pH through moisturization is still in development, ceramide-dominant emollients and medical devices have become available in the effort to restore the lipid imbalance in atopic skin. Discoveries in the near future of specific ceramide groups that are deficient and play a role in AD should further refine therapeutic intervention. Given that ceramides regulate keratinocyte differentiation, proliferation and apoptosis (and do not just provide 'mortar' between keratinocytes as a physical barrier), modulation of epidermal ceramides may also impact the inflammation and skin thickening of AD.

The Importance of *Staphylococcus aureus* in Atopic Dermatitis

The skin of patients with AD is inherently favorable for *Staphylococcus aureus* colonization. In contrast to a prevalence of a carrier state in 5–20% of nonatopic individuals, *S. aureus* is recovered in approximately 90% of patients from lesions of AD, 76% from uninvolved (normal) skin and approximately 80% from the anterior nares. The increased adherence of *S. aureus* to the epidermal cells of individuals with AD has been attributed to exposure of extracellular matrix components such as fibronectin through scratching and a poor epidermal barrier, which is likely perpetuated by ceramidases and neuraminidases elaborated by the staphylococci. Bacterial colonization likely relates as well to a markedly diminished production of endogenous antimicrobial peptides in the inflamed skin of patients with AD [16]. Staphylococcal infection has clearly been demonstrated to exacerbate inflammation, and several mechanisms have been proposed. *S. aureus* release superantigen toxins that have been shown to trigger inflammation, in part through activating superantigen-specific and allergen-specific T cells and leading to release of IL-31, a cytokine linked to pruritus. However, superantigen is not the only exacerbant of the inflammation. In fact, production of superantigen does not necessarily correlate with an increase in EASI (Eczema Area and Severity Index) score or lesional cytokines [17]. A recent study has shown that concentrations of lipoteichoic acid, a bacterial lipoprotein, correlate with EASI score and increase epidermal cytokines when injected into skin [18]. Poor response to traditional topical therapy in the face of staphylococcal infection has been attributed to the shift, induced by bacteria, to an alternatively spliced glucocorticoid receptor which prevents corticosteroid binding to T cells. These observations emphasize the role of *S. aureus* as an important trigger of AD and endorse therapies that decrease the numbers of bacteria on the skin (see below). Indeed, decades of anecdotal experience has shown that treatment of secondary infection with antibiotics improves the skin inflammation in addition to areas of infection, although a recent meta-analysis found no good study to test this observation scientifically [19]. Although methicillin-resistant *S. aureus* colonization and superinfection of AD is increasing, the majority of children with AD harbor methicillin-sensitive *S. aureus*. Nevertheless, avoidance of unnecessary antibiotic therapy in patients with AD is advisable, especially given the greater difficulty in treating infection in patients with methicillin-resistant *S. aureus*.

Improving Atopic Dermatitis through Decreasing Organisms

Nonantibiotic antiseptics are a potential means to decrease bacterial overload without increasing resistance of organisms to antibiotics. In general, studies have not been successful and suggest that almost total-body exposure is necessary to be effective. Most promising has been studies with dilute sodium hypochlorite (bleach) in the bathwater. A single-blind, randomized controlled trial of sodium hypochlorite 0.005% twice weekly with intranasal mupirocin monthly for 5 days was performed in children with infected, moderate-to-severe AD. All children were treated initially with cephalexin, but the baths and intranasal application (or placebo) were continued for 3 months. Within 3 months after initiation, patients treated with dilute bleach baths showed a significant decrease in the percentage of patients with specified IGA (Investigator's Global Assessment) scores, difference in EASI score (including after adjustment for baseline differences between groups), and body surface area affected [20]. Interestingly, bath submerged sites (limbs and trunk), but not bath exposed sites (head and neck) showed the improvement, suggesting that the baths rather than the intranasal mupirocin treatment, played the major role in causing improvement. Dilute bleach baths have been well tolerated, although when skin is raw because of infection, a short period of improvement may be required before bath initiation. The failure to clear *S. aureus* with bath treatment emphasizes the need for continuing baths as maintenance therapy, but it should be noted that no quantification to prove reduction of the *S. aureus* was performed in this trial.

Keratinocytes produce proinflammatory cytokines and antimicrobial peptides (β-defensins, cathelicidins) in response to Toll-like receptor stimulation by injury and organisms. In patients with AD, the antimicrobial response is dampened [16], although not as a primary defect but rather because of the presence of Th2 cytokines [21]. Vitamin D_3 upregulates the expression of cathelicidin, including in the skin of individuals with AD [22, 23]. Topical application, however, is too irritating and has been shown to increase keratinocyte production of TSLP [23]. Daily oral administration of 4,000 IU of vitamin D_3 for 21 days induced cathelicidin expression in lesional skin [22]. In addition, a small pilot study of ergocalciferol 1,000 IU/day for 1 month led to a significantly greater decrease in IGA score, although patients had mild AD

[24]. Studies to evaluate the potential for supplemental vitamin D_3 as an adjunctive therapy for AD are ongoing.

Topical Anti-inflammatory Therapy Continues to Be Critical as Treatment

Topically applied corticosteroids have been the mainstay of AD therapy for decades. Concern about potential toxicity, especially local side effects at sensitive sites and with chronic use, has promoted the utilization of calcineurin inhibitors (topically applied tacrolimus ointment and pimecrolimus cream) as steroid-sparing agents. Indeed, topically applied corticosteroids have recently been shown within 2–3 days of application to decrease epidermal proliferation and differentiation, decrease lipid synthesis and increase kallikrein 7 expression [25]. Calcineurin inhibitors have now been available for more than a decade commercially and are establishing a track record of safety. Given the new focus on epidermal barrier, one question is whether calcineurin inhibitors could reverse the barrier defect of steroids. Pimecrolimus treatment was recently shown to improve the lipid barrier in comparison with application of betamethasone valerate [26].

Almost a decade ago, maintenance therapy with twice weekly application of fluticasone was shown to decrease dermatitis relapses. More recently, this principle has been applied to utilization of topical calcineurin inhibitors in an effort to test a rotational use of topical steroids and calcineurin inhibitors, thereby limiting the chronic utilization of either type of medication. Studies in Europe and the United States have shown that 2–3 times weekly application of tacrolimus ointment to recurrently flaring areas during periods of good control reduces flares overall and the requirement for topical corticosteroid application [27, 28]. In fact, twice weekly maintenance therapy is now an approved indication in Europe in treating AD.

A continuing concern, however, is the Black Box warning issued by the US Food and Drug Administration about the use of calcineurin inhibitors in 2006. Despite lack of evidence of systemic absorption from topical application of these medications, this warning was based on a theoretical concern of increased cancer risk from the experience of systemic administration in transplant patients and animal studies with administration of high concentrations. To date, there is no signal of an increased risk. In fact, in a questionnaire study, the OR of association with nonmelanoma skin cancer in 5,000 adults with AD decreased as the number of tubes and potency of topical calcineurin inhibitors increased [29]. Furthermore, the risk of lymphoma has not been shown to increase with use either [30]. On the other hand, these studies from both the UK and the US demonstrated a clear association between risk of lymphoma and severity of the AD [31]. Ongoing long-term studies of the use of pimecrolimus cream, including in infants, and tacrolimus ointment for AD have disclosed no evidence of increased occurrence of lymphoma or nonmelanoma skin cancer to date.

The Recalcitrant Patient

Despite the best efforts at trigger avoidance, proper bathing and moisturizing, use of anti-inflammatory topical medications and treatment of secondary infection, patients may not respond. In these cases, it is always important to consider poor compliance. Using stealth monitoring through electronic caps, Krejci-Manwaring et al. [32] showed that only 32% of patients with AD were compliant with twice daily application during 8 weeks of observation, and suggest that many patients deemed to have tachyphylaxis to topical steroids are poorly compliant. The clinician must take the time to properly educate and ensure that the patient and family understand the reasons and need for the prescribed therapy. Exploring the reasons for poor compliance may lead to a new regimen that can more easily be followed and, thus, successful. In other patients, the apparent failure to respond may, instead, reflect secondary contact dermatitis to a topical agent used for AD. In recent studies, 6.2–22% of children with AD showed positive patch tests for potential allergens other than nickel, a common cause of periumbilical exacerbation of dermatitis. In one study, half of these children showed reactivity to their emollient with a variety of individual ingredients found to the responsible (avena extract, wheat protein, calendula, lanolin); others showed reactivity to topical antiseptic (chlorhexidine) and one to the topical steroid [33]. Other patients may have a significant allergic trigger that has been missed, requiring careful evaluation of history and possibly additional allergy testing to discover the culprit.

In severely affected patients with AD, topical therapy is insufficient. Phototherapy may be the first choice because of safety, but may be poorly tolerated as initial therapy if the skin is highly inflamed, and is often alternatively chosen as maintenance therapy. For many families, the time demands of phototherapy cannot be met, especially with a busy lifestyle and if far from a therapeutic center. If the impact on quality of life for the patient and family is severely impacted by the inflammatory skin disorder, systemic immunosuppressant therapy is an important consideration. While to date biologic therapy has not found success in individuals with AD as has been seen with psoriasis, most severely affected patients show responses to cyclosporine, azathioprine, mycophenolate mofetil or methotrexate. No comparative trials have yet been undertaken with systemic therapy, especially in pediatric patients, and guidelines for duration of utilization are needed.

Conclusions

Recent discoveries have refocused attention on barrier defects in AD as a primary problem, including in the development of the atopic march. The interplay between immune abnormalities and barrier dysfunction blur the distinction between 'extrinsic' and 'intrinsic' AD, suggesting that these terms be abandoned. Current therapies should learn from our recent discoveries, and be directed towards decreasing inflammation, improving the epidermal barrier and decreasing bacterial colonization/infection, one of the most common triggers in patients with moderate-to-severe disease. Future therapies may be: (1) more targeted towards an individual's gene defect(s), such as means to increase filaggrin expression; (2) suppression of protease activation; (3) targeting AD-specific proinflammatory molecules, such as by blocking TSLP function, or activated signaling, such as with topical NF-κB decoys; (4) increasing production of antimicrobial peptides, such as through oral vitamin D_3; and (5) decreasing the sensation of pruritus, such as through blockade of IL-31 expression or function.

References

1 Spergel JM, Paller AS: Atopic dermatitis and the atopic march. J Allergy Clin Immunol 2003;112:S118–S127.

2 Bieber T, Novak N: Pathogenesis of atopic dermatitis: new developments. Curr Allergy Asthma Rep 2009;9:291–294.

3 Elias PM, Steinhoff M: 'Outside-to-inside' (and now back to 'outside') pathogenic mechanisms in atopic dermatitis. J Invest Dermatol 2008;128:1067–1070.

4 Palmer CN, Irvine AD, Terron-Kwiatkowski A, Zhao Y, Liao H, Lee SP, Goudie DR, Sandilands A, Campbell LE, Smith FJ, O'Regan GM, Watson RM, Cecil JE, Bale SJ, Compton JG, DiGiovanna JJ, Fleckman P, Lewis-Jones S, Arseculeratne G, Sergeant A, Munro CS, El Houate B, McElreavey K, Halkjaer LB, Bisgaard H, Mukhopadhyay S, McLean WH: Common loss-of-function variants of the epidermal barrier protein filaggrin are a major predisposing factor for atopic dermatitis. Nat Genet 2006;38:441–446.

5 van den Oord RA, Sheikh A: Filaggrin gene defects and risk of developing allergic sensitisation and allergic disorders: systematic review and meta-analysis. BMJ 2009;339:b2433.

6 Howell MD, Kim BE, Gao P, Grant AV, Boguniewicz M, DeBenedetto A, Schneider L, Beck LA, Barnes KC, Leung DY: Cytokine modulation of atopic dermatitis filaggrin skin expression. J Allergy Clin Immunol 2009;124:R7–R12.

7 Broccardo CJ, Mahaffey S, Schwarz J, Wruck L, David G, Schlievert PM, Reisdorph NA, Leung DY: Comparative proteomic profiling of patients with atopic dermatitis based on history of eczema herpeticum infection and *Staphylococcus aureus* colonization. J Allergy Clin Immunol 2011;127:186–193, 193.e181–111.

8 Voegeli R, Rawlings AV, Breternitz M, Doppler S, Schreier T, Fluhr JW: Increased stratum corneum serine protease activity in acute eczematous atopic skin. Br J Dermatol 2009;161:70–77.

9 Briot A, Deraison C, Lacroix M, Bonnart C, Robin A, Besson C, Dubus P, Hovnanian A: Kallikrein 5 induces atopic dermatitis-like lesions through PAR2-mediated thymic stromal lymphopoietin expression in Netherton syndrome. J Exp Med 2009;206:1135–1147.

10 Oyoshi MK, Larson RP, Ziegler SF, Geha RS: Mechanical injury polarizes skin dendritic cells to elicit a T(H)2 response by inducing cutaneous thymic stromal lymphopoietin expression. J Allergy Clin Immunol 2010;126:976–984, 984.e1–5.

11 Demehri S, Morimoto M, Holtzman MJ, Kopan R: Skin-derived TSLP triggers progression from epidermal-barrier defects to asthma. PLoS Biol 2009;7:e1000067.

12 Imokawa G: A possible mechanism underlying the ceramide deficiency in atopic dermatitis: expression of a deacylase enzyme that cleaves the N-acyl linkage of sphingomyelin and glucosylceramide. J Dermatol Sci 2009;55:1–9.

13 Ishikawa J, Narita H, Kondo N, Hotta M, Takagi Y, Masukawa Y, Kitahara T, Takema Y, Koyano S, Yamazaki S, Hatamochi A: Changes in the ceramide profile of atopic dermatitis patients. J Invest Dermatol 2010;130:2511–2514.

14 Jungersted JM, Scheer H, Mempel M, Baurecht H, Cifuentes L, Hogh JK, Hellgren LI, Jemec GB, Agner T, Weidinger S: Stratum corneum lipids, skin barrier function and filaggrin mutations in patients with atopic eczema. Allergy 2010;65:911–918.

15 Hatano Y, Man MQ, Uchida Y, Crumrine D, Scharschmidt TC, Kim EG, Mauro TM, Feingold KR, Elias PM, Holleran WM: Maintenance of an acidic stratum corneum prevents emergence of murine atopic dermatitis. J Invest Dermatol 2009;129:1824–1835.

16 Ong PY, Ohtake T, Brandt C, Strickland I, Boguniewicz M, Ganz T, Gallo RL, Leung DY: Endogenous antimicrobial peptides and skin infections in atopic dermatitis. N Engl J Med 2002;347:1151–1160.

17 Kozman A, Yao Y, Bina P, Saha C, Yao W, Kaplan MH, Travers JB: Encoding a superantigen by *Staphylococcus aureus* does not affect clinical characteristics of infected atopic dermatitis lesions. Br J Dermatol 2010;163:1308–1311.
18 Travers JB, Kozman A, Mousdicas N, Saha C, Landis M, Al-Hassani M, Yao W, Yao Y, Hyatt AM, Sheehan MP, Haggstrom AN, Kaplan MH: Infected atopic dermatitis lesions contain pharmacologic amounts of lipoteichoic acid. J Allergy Clin Immunol 2010; 125:146–152.e1–2.
19 Birnie AJ, Bath-Hextall FJ, Ravenscroft JC, Williams HC: Interventions to reduce *Staphylococcus aureus* in the management of atopic eczema. Cochrane Database Syst Rev 2008:CD003871.
20 Huang JT, Abrams M, Tlougan B, Rademaker A, Paller AS: Treatment of *Staphylococcus aureus* colonization in atopic dermatitis decreases disease severity. Pediatrics 2009;123:e808–e814.
21 Nomura I, Goleva E, Howell MD, Hamid QA, Ong PY, Hall CF, Darst MA, Gao B, Boguniewicz M, Travers JB, Leung DY: Cytokine milieu of atopic dermatitis, as compared to psoriasis, skin prevents induction of innate immune response genes. J Immunol 2003;171:3262–3269.
22 Hata TR, Kotol P, Jackson M, Nguyen M, Paik A, Udall D, Kanada K, Yamasaki K, Alexandrescu D, Gallo RL: Administration of oral vitamin D induces cathelicidin production in atopic individuals. J Allergy Clin Immunol 2008;122:829–831.
23 Li M, Hener P, Zhang Z, Ganti KP, Metzger D, Chambon P: Induction of thymic stromal lymphopoietin expression in keratinocytes is necessary for generating an atopic dermatitis upon application of the active vitamin D_3 analogue MC903 on mouse skin. J Invest Dermatol 2009;129:498–502.
24 Sidbury R, Sullivan AF, Thadhani RI, Camargo CA Jr: Randomized controlled trial of vitamin D supplementation for winter-related atopic dermatitis in Boston: a pilot study. Br J Dermatol 2008;159: 245–247.
25 Cork MJ, Danby SG, Vasilopoulos Y, Hadgraft J, Lane ME, Moustafa M, Guy RH, Macgowan AL, Tazi-Ahnini R, Ward SJ: Epidermal barrier dysfunction in atopic dermatitis. J Invest Dermatol 2009;129: 1892–1908.
26 Jensen JM, Pfeiffer S, Witt M, Brautigam M, Neumann C, Weichenthal M, Schwarz T, Folster-Holst R, Proksch E: Different effects of pimecrolimus and betamethasone on the skin barrier in patients with atopic dermatitis. J Allergy Clin Immunol 2009;123:1124–1133.
27 Paller AS, Eichenfield LF, Kirsner RS, Shull T, Jaracz E, Simpson EL: Three times weekly tacrolimus ointment reduces relapse in stabilized atopic dermatitis: a new paradigm for use. Pediatrics 2008;122: e1210–e1218.
28 Breneman D, Fleischer AB Jr, Abramovits W, Zeichner J, Gold MH, Kirsner RS, Shull TF, Crowe AW, Jaracz E, Hanifin JM: Intermittent therapy for flare prevention and long-term disease control in stabilized atopic dermatitis: a randomized comparison of 3-times-weekly applications of tacrolimus ointment versus vehicle. J Am Acad Dermatol 2008; 58:990–999.
29 Margolis DJ, Hoffstad O, Bilker W: Lack of association between exposure to topical calcineurin inhibitors and skin cancer in adults. Dermatology 2007; 214:289–295.
30 Arellano FM, Wentworth CE, Arana A, Fernandez C, Paul CF: Risk of lymphoma following exposure to calcineurin inhibitors and topical steroids in patients with atopic dermatitis. J Invest Dermatol 2007;127:808–816.
31 Arana A, Wentworth CE, Fernandez-Vidaurre C, Schlienger RG, Conde E, Arellano FM: Incidence of cancer in the general population and in patients with or without atopic dermatitis in the U.K. Br J Dermatol 2010;163:1036–1043.
32 Krejci-Manwaring J, Tusa MG, Carroll C, Camacho F, Kaur M, Carr D, Fleischer AB Jr: Balkrishnan R, Feldman SR: Stealth monitoring of adherence to topical medication: adherence is very poor in children with atopic dermatitis. J Am Acad Dermatol 2007;56:211–216.
33 Mailhol C, Lauwers-Cances V, Rance F, Paul C, Giordano-Labadie F: Prevalence and risk factors for allergic contact dermatitis to topical treatment in atopic dermatitis: a study in 641 children. Allergy 2009;64:801–806.

Dr. Amy S. Paller
Department of Dermatology, Northwestern University Feinberg School of Medicine
676 N. St. Clair Street, Suite 1600
Chicago, IL 60611-2941 (USA)
Tel. +1 312 695 3721, E-Mail apaller@northwestern.edu

Author Index

Subject Index